atlas of
CHEST infections

Dr Margaret E. Hodson
MD, MSc, FRCP, DA
Reader in Respiratory Medicine
Honorary Consultant Physician
National Heart and Lung Institute
The Royal Brompton Hospital, London

Dr Ian D. Starke
MD, MSc, MRCP
Consultant Physician and Senior Lecturer in
Medicine for the Elderly
Lewisham Hospital and UMDS, Guy's Campus
London

Professor Bryan Corrin
MD, FRCPath
Professor of Thoracic Pathology
National Heart and Lung Institute
The Royal Brompton Hospital, London

Dr Ian H. Kerr
MA, MBBChir, FRCP, FRCR
Honorary Consulting Radiologist
The Royal Brompton Hospital, London

Professor Dame Margaret Turner-Warwick
DBE, DM, PhD, DSc(Hon), FRCP(E), FRACP, FACP, FFOM, PRCP
President
Royal College of Physicians, London

GOWER MEDICAL PUBLISHING · LONDON · NEW YORK

Distributed in the USA and Canada by:
Raven Press Ltd.
1185 Avenue of the Americas
New York
New York 10036
USA

Distributed in the rest of the world by:
Gower Medical Publishing
Middlesex house
34-42 Cleveland Street
London W1P 5FB
UK

British Library Cataloguing in Publication Data:
available on request

**Library of Congress Cataloging in Publication
Data:** available on request

ISBN 1-56375-553-X

Publisher: Michele Campbell

Project Manager: Alison Whitehouse

Layout Design: Caroline Archer

Cover Design: Balvir Koura

Index: Nina Boyd

Production: Susan Bishop

Typeset by M to N Typesetters, London
Text and legends set in Palatino

Originated by Mandarin,Hong Kong

Produced by Mandarin Offset (HK) Ltd
Printed and bound in Hong Kong.

Preface

This atlas illustrates pulmonary infections due to a variety of microorganisms. A special section has been devoted to tuberculosis. As the incidence of tuberculosis declines, it is particularly important that doctors are familiar with its multiple radiological appearances so that they make the correct diagnosis when the disease presents. Throughout the atlas the particular problems of diagnosing infection in the immunosuppressed patient have been highlighted. These patients are increasing in numbers due to increased organ transplantation and the AIDS epidemic.

The material in this book is derived from *Clinical Atlas of Respiratory Diseases* by Margaret Turner-Warwick, Margaret Hodson, Bryan Corrin and Ian Kerr (Gower Medical Publishing, 1989). It is not a textbook and should be read in conjunction with an up-to-date textbook of respiratory medicine in which, of necessity, illustration will be limited. Undergraduates, postgraduate students and practising consultants will we hope find this atlas helpful.

We are extremely grateful to a large number of people who have helped us to compile the material for this atlas; we hope our acknowledgements are complete and apologise if there are any omissions. We would like to thank our medical publishers and the project editor for their assistance in this venture.

MARGARET E. HODSON
IAN D. STARKE
BRYAN CORRIN
IAN H. KERR
MARGARET TURNER-WARWICK

Contents

Chapter 1

Introduction

INTRODUCTION

Pneumonia may be defined as inflammation in the lung parenchyma. Consolidation is said to occur when the alveolar air is replaced by an exudate and there is airlessness without shrinkage. Pneumonia can be classified anatomically as lobar pneumonia or bronchopneumonia. In lobar pneumonia (Figs 1.1 and 1.2), areas of uniform consolidation are present in a lobe, or lobes, of the lung; in bronchopneumonia the consolidation is patchy, multifocal and often bilateral (Figs 1.3–1.5).

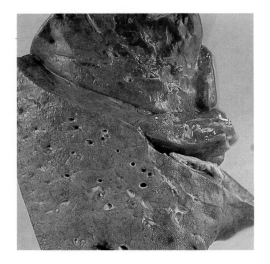

FIGURE 1.1 Pneumococcal lobar pneumonia. The lower lobe is pale and uniformly consolidated and has not collapsed on slicing as the upper and middle lobes have done.

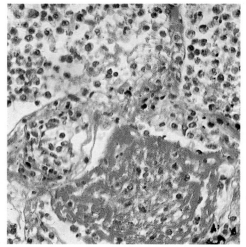
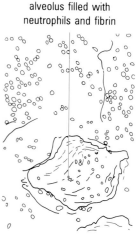

alveolus filled with neutrophils and fibrin

FIGURE 1.2 Pneumococcal lobar pneumonia. The alveoli are consolidated by an exudate of neutrophil polymorphonuclear leucocytes and fibrin, contracted into discrete knots. Haematoxylin and eosin stain.

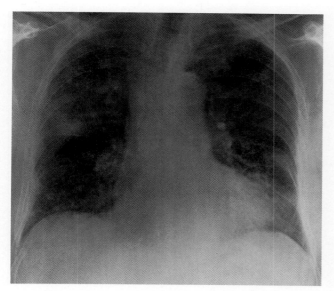

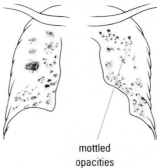

mottled
opacities

FIGURE 1.3 Bronchopneumonia.
Ill-defined opacities of various
sizes are present in both lungs.

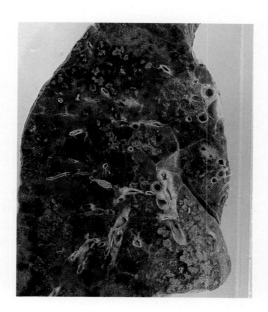

FIGURE 1.4 Bronchopneumonia.
Foci of peribronchiolar
consolidation are surrounded
by congestion.

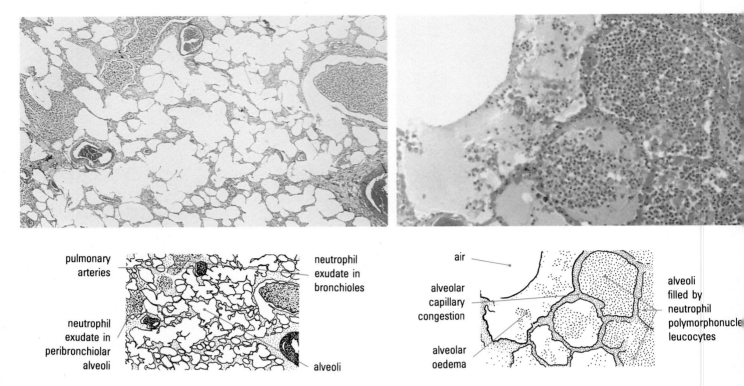

pulmonary arteries

neutrophil exudate in bronchioles

neutrophil exudate in peribronchiolar alveoli

alveoli

air

alveolar capillary congestion

alveolar oedema

alveoli filled by neutrophil polymorphonuclear leucocytes

FIGURE 1.5   Bronchopneumonia. The low-power photomicrograph (left) represents an early stage. Much of the acute inflammatory exudate is still within conductive airways but there is some extension into peribronchiolar alveoli. Higher magnification (right) shows neutrophils filling several alveoli, capillary congestion and alveolar oedema. The latter may have occurred first and predisposed to infection (hypostatic pneumonia). Haematoxylin and eosin stain.

Since the decline in incidence of acute pneumococcal lobar pneumonia with the introduction of antibiotics, it is probably more helpful to classify pneumonia according to aetiology (Fig. 1.6) rather than anatomical distribution.

Pneumonia is usually caused by microorganisms such as bacteria, viruses, chlamydia, mycoplasma, rickettsias, fungi or protozoa. The term pneumonitis is synonymous with pneumonia but is often preferentially used when the cause of inflammation is non-infective, for example an allergic reaction or chemical or physical injury.

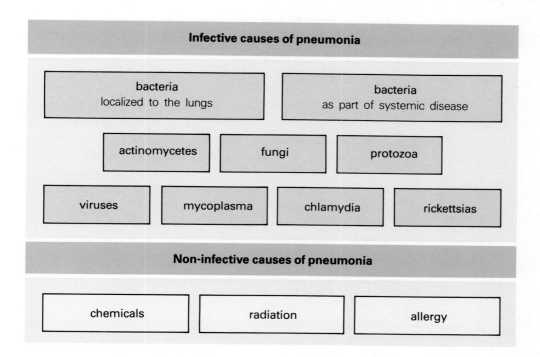

FIGURE 1.6 Aetiology of pneumonia.

PREDISPOSING FACTORS

Pneumonia is most commonly found among the very young, the very old and people suffering from other diseases, such as diabetes mellitus, alcoholism, malignant disease or immune deficiency due to drugs or disease. Patients with pre-existing lung disease such as bronchitis, bronchiectasis, cystic fibrosis or carcinoma of the lung are particularly prone to develop pneumonia. Patients with upper respiratory tract infections including sinusitis, those with diseases of the oesophagus, postsurgical patients and those who smoke also have an increased risk of pneumonia. Bacterial pneumonias often follow viral infection such as influenza. Other predisposing factors include obstruction of the airways by foreign bodies or carcinoma and the aspiration of vomit.

These predisposing factors all act by causing impairment of one or more host defence mechanisms. These may be localized (e.g. a foreign body) or generalized (e.g. patients with severe malnutrition), and range from mild (e.g. old age) to severe (e.g. patients undergoing bone marrow transplantation). The probability of developing pneumonia, the severity and rapidity of its progress, and the range of possible causative organisms all increase with increasingly severe impairment of host defence (immunocompromise).

The term 'opportunistic infection' may be defined as one in which an organism that would not be expected to infect a normal individual becomes able to cause infection because of some impairment in host defence mechanisms. It is an imprecise term that is also used to describe an increase in the severity of an infection in those who are immunocompromised. The different uses of the term serve only to illustrate the difficulties in drawing precise boundaries in this rather indistinct area.

MORTALITY

Mortality from pneumonia in young and middle-aged adults who were previously fit is now very low. There was a tremendous drop in mortality with the advent of penicillin and over the last twenty years the death rate of UK infants with pneumonia has continued to decline. The commonest causes of pneumonia in the very young are respiratory syncytial virus and staphylococcus, the latter responding well to appropriate antibiotics.

The incidence of pneumonia in the very old is increasing in the United Kingdom. This is probably because, with improving medical and social conditions, more people are living to old age. Pneumonia is commonly a terminal event in the elderly and is frequently entered on death certificates. At all ages the death rate in males is higher than in females.

Chapter 2

Bacterial Pneumonias

BACTERIAL PNEUMONIAS

Some of the bacteria which cause pneumonia are illustrated in Figs 2.1 and 2.2. *Streptococcus pneumoniae* (also called pneumococcus) is the commonest cause of acute bacterial pneumonia in previously healthy young adults. The onset is characteristically sudden with a high pyrexia, rigor, pleuritic chest pain and cough. Within a few hours, rust-coloured sputum is produced; herpes labialis is a common accompanying feature. At this stage, the patient may appear flushed with a high respiration rate and pleuritic chest pain. If the infection is severe there may be cyanosis and hypotension. The early physical signs in the chest are:

1. Diminished expansion
2. Impaired percussion note
3. Diminished normal breath sounds
4. Crepitations.

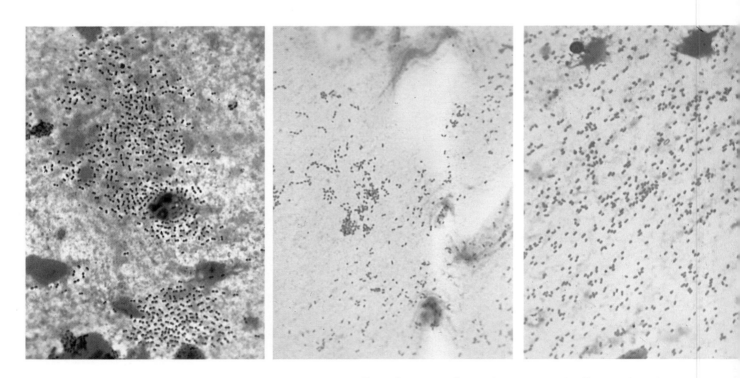

FIGURE 2.1 Bacteria commonly causing pneumonia. Gram stains of sputum showing capsulated Gram-positive cocci of *Streptococcus pneumoniae* (left), small Gram-negative bacilli of *Haemophilus influenzae* (centre) and Gram-negative bacilli of *Pseudomonas aeruginosa* (right). Courtesy of Dr H. Gaya.

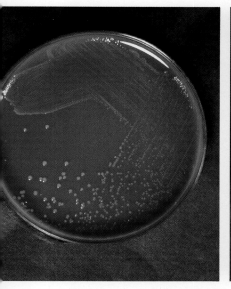 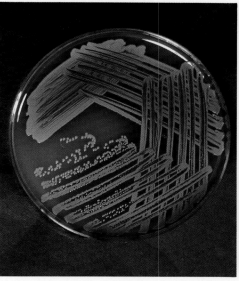 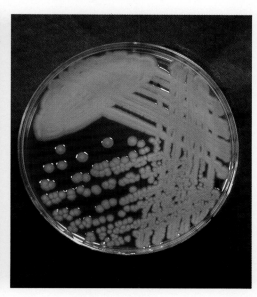

FIGURE 2.2 Bacteria commonly causing pneumonia. Cultures of *Haemophilus influenzae* (18 hours, 7% chocolate agar; left), *Staphylococcus aureus* (18 hours, 7% blood agar; centre) and *Klebsiella pneumoniae* (18 hours, MacConkey's agar; right). Courtesy of Dr H. Gaya.

After a further 24–36 hours, consolidation occurs and the physical signs are:

1. Diminished expansion
2. Dull percussion note
3. High-pitched bronchial breathing
4. Increased tactile vocal fremitus and whispering pectoriloquy
5. Widespread crepitations
6. A pleural rub is sometimes present.

If the patient develops complications such as a pleural effusion or areas of collapse, the physical signs will vary.

Chest radiographs show lobar consolidation (Fig. 2.3). The white blood count is characteristically high and the organism can be isolated from the sputum and often also from blood cultures. The disease responds well to treatment with benzyl penicillin.

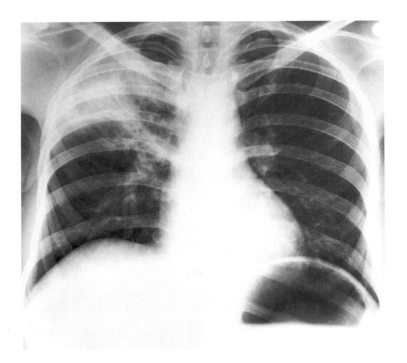

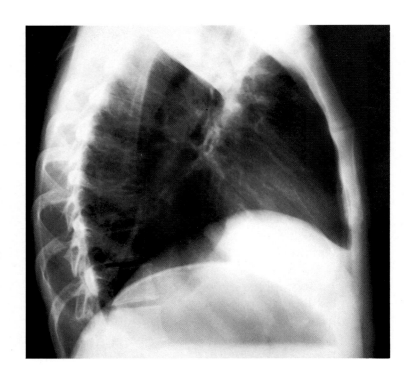

FIGURE 2.3   Pneumococcal pneumonia. There is dense homogenous opacification of the right upper lobe, mainly the posterior segment. Note the air bronchogram indicating solid lung with patent airways. The patient developed sudden onset of cough and pleuritic chest pain; he had herpes simplex on his lips, a temperature of 39.9°C and a white cell count of $20 \times 10^9/l$. *Streptococcus pneumoniae* was isolated from sputum and blood culture.

Pneumonia due to *Staphylococcus pyogenes* may be found among patients who are debilitated, immuno-suppressed or have some other focus of staphylococcal infection. Cases also occur following influenza epidemics (Figs 2.4 and 2.5). Pneumonia is often severe and cavities may form. Treatment is with antibiotics to which the pathogen is sensitive; these may include flucloxacillin, erythromycin, lincomycin, clindamycin or sodium fusidate.

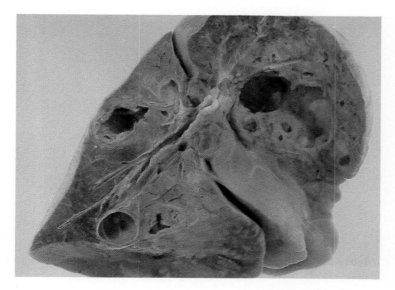

FIGURE 2.4 Staphylococcal pneumonia. Pneumatoceles resulted from staphylococcal lung abscesses in this child.

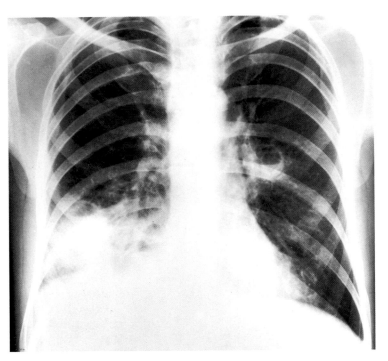

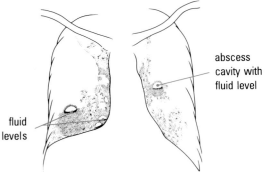

FIGURE 2.5 Staphylococcal pneumonia. There is consolidation at the right base and thin-walled cavities with fluid levels at the right base and left mid-zone.

Infection with *Haemophilus influenzae* is usually found in patients with pre-existing lung disease and will respond to a variety of antibiotics such as ampicillin, amoxycillin, tetracycline, the cephalosporins or co-trimoxazole.

Klebsiella pneumoniae can cause extensive consolidation and is often found in people with pre-existing lung diseases (Figs 2.6 and 2.7). It is usually treated with chloramphenicol and aminoglycoside.

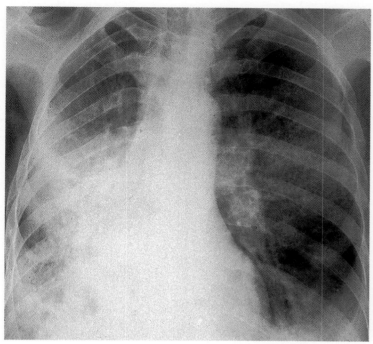

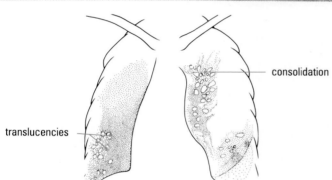

FIGURE 2.6 Klebsiella pneumonia. Widespread consolidation occurs, with small areas of translucency. There is an element of collapse of the right lung, indicated by mediastinal shift. A small left pleural effusion is present. This middle-aged patient was extremely ill and required a period of artificial ventilation in addition to antibiotics.

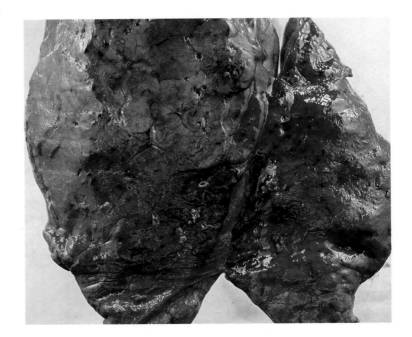

FIGURE 2.7 Klebsiella pneumonia. There is confluent lobular consolidation in the upper part of the upper lobe. The boundary between consolidated and normal lung is across the lobe and not at an interlobar fissure as in true lobar pneumonia.

Other causes of bacterial pneumonia are *Streptococcus pyogenes*, *Escherichia coli*, *Pseudomonas aeruginosa* and *Bacteroides*. Infection with Gram-negative organisms, particularly *Pseudomonas aeruginosa*, is often found among patients with pre-existing lung disease, such as bronchiectasis or cystic fibrosis. Other groups particularly at risk are those with diabetes mellitus, alcoholism or impaired immune defences and those receiving mechanical ventilation. Infection with *P. aeruginosa* will usually respond to treatment with anti-pseudomonal penicillins or cephalosporins and aminoglycosides. Where facilities are available, the dose of aminoglycoside should be regulated according to serum levels. Infection with anaerobes (Figs 2.8 and 2.9) will respond to metronidazole, penicillin, chloramphenicol and other antibiotics active against the particular organism.

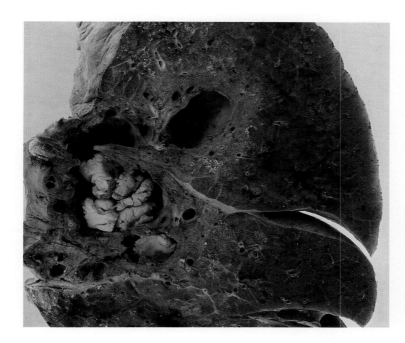

FIGURE 2.8 Primary lung abscesses containing inspissated pus. The abscesses involve the sites of predilection of aspiration lesions, the apical segment of the lower lobe and the posterior segment of the upper lobe.

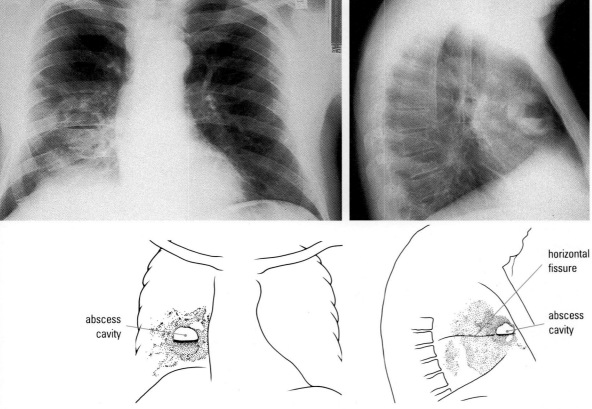

FIGURE 2.9 Anaerobic abscess due to *Bacteroides fragilis*. There is a 3cm abscess cavity with fluid level and some patchy surrounding consolidation in the anterior segment of the right upper lobe and middle lobe. This might easily be mistaken for a carcinoma.

Legionella pneumophilia was first described in 1976 after an outbreak among American legionnaires in Philadelphia. It is now realized that this type of pneumonia can occur in a mild form, but some outbreaks have shown a high mortality.

Many systemic features such as headache, confusion, abdominal pain and diarrhoea occur, in addition to pulmonary symptoms such as cough and pleuritic chest pain. There is often leucopenia, associated hyponatraemia and albuminuria.

There is nothing specific about the pathology (Figs 2.10 and 2.11). The pathogen is recognized on electron

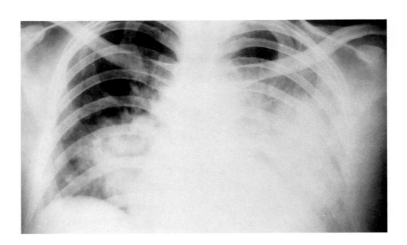

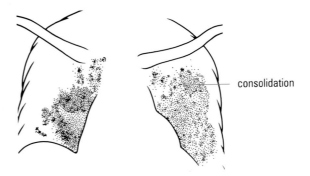

FIGURE 2.10 Legionnaires' pneumonia. Ill-defined areas of opacification are seen in both lungs, but particularly the left.

consolidation

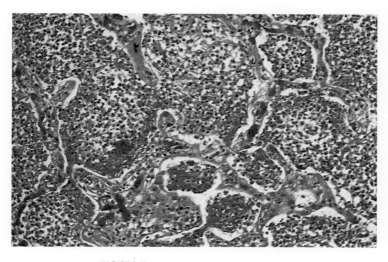

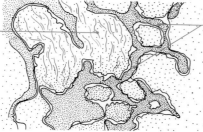

alveoli filled by
a fibrinous and
neutrophil
exudate

interalveolar
septa

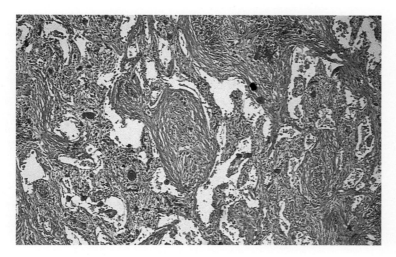

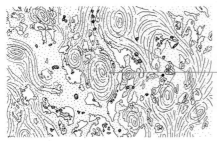

whorled knots
of collagen
fill the
alveoli

FIGURE 2.11 Legionnaires'
pneumonia. The alveoli are
consolidated by a fibrin and
neutrophil exudate (upper),
changes resembling those seen
in pneumococcal lobar
pneumonia. Healing has
occurred by fibrosis rather than
resolution (lower). The scarring
is mainly intra-alveolar.
Haematoxylin and eosin stain.

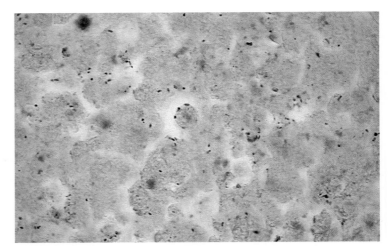

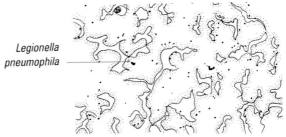

Legionella
pneumophila

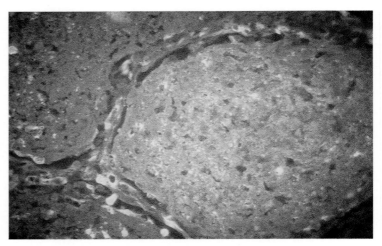

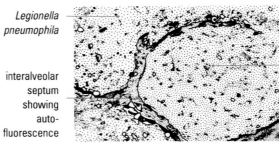

Legionella
pneumophila

interalveolar
septum
showing
auto-
fluorescence

background
staining
represents
bacterial
antigen

FIGURE 2.12   Legionnaires'
pneumonia. Bacteria are
detected in the alveolar exudate
using Dieterle's silver stain
(upper). Immunofluorescent
microscopy is used to identify
the causative organism:
Legionella pneumophila (lower).

microscopy, immunofluorescent microscopy or by Dieterle staining of a lung section (Figs 2.12 and 2.13). The diagnosis may also be made by serological testing, where an antibody titre of 1:256 or greater, or a four-fold rise in titre, is considered to be diagnostic. The most effective treatment appears to be erythromycin plus rifampicin.

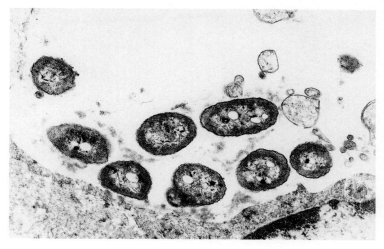

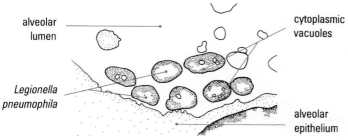

FIGURE 2.13 Legionnaires' pneumonia. The electronmicrograph shows the fine detail of the causative organisms, which resemble other coccobacilli.

Bacterial pneumonia may also accompany a systemic bacterial disease such as pertussis, typhoid, brucellosis, plague (Figs 2.14 and 2.15) or anthrax.

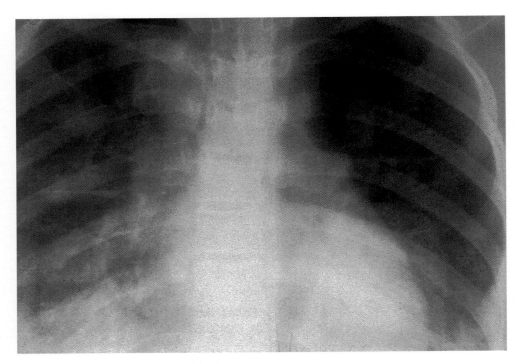

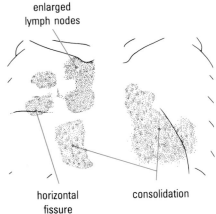

FIGURE 2.14 Pulmonary involvement in bubonic plague. Infection of the lungs is via the blood. There are enlarged hilar and paratracheal lymph nodes with patchy consolidation in both lungs.

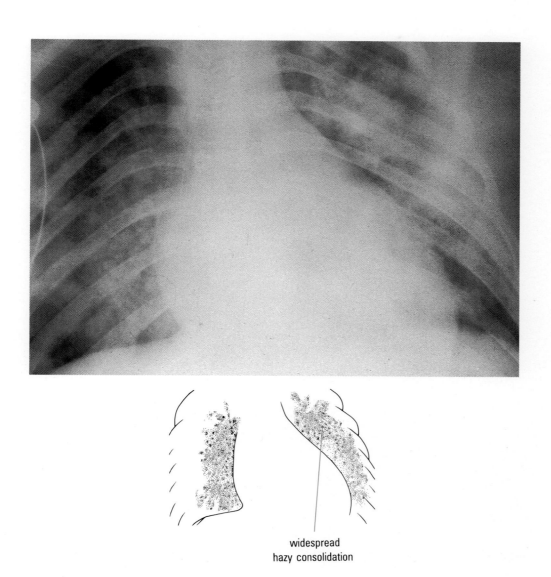

widespread
hazy consolidation

FIGURE 2.15 Pneumonic plague. Infection is by inhalation.
Consolidation is widespread and an air bronchogram is present.

Chapter 3

Tuberculosis

Tuberculosis has been a scourge of mankind throughout history. Although the number of cases in the developed world is now rapidly decreasing, it is still a major problem in the developing countries. A survey in 1971 in rural Vietnam showed that 0.7 percent of the population had positive sputum on direct smear testing. The World Health Organization estimates that there are

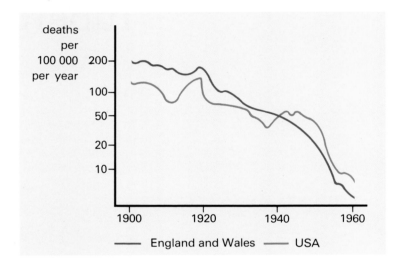

FIGURE 3.1   Deaths from tuberculosis between 1900 and 1960 in England and Wales, and the USA.

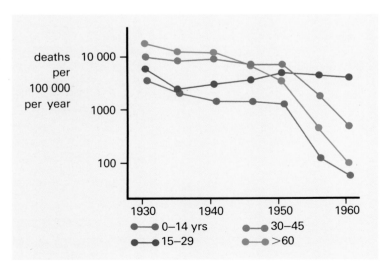

FIGURE 3.2   Deaths from tuberculosis during the period 1930–1960 according to age group.

about 15–20 million cases of tuberculosis in the world at any one time, with about three million deaths per year. There were so many deaths in the United Kingdom in the eighteenth century that the disease was known as the 'white plague'. The incidence had begun to decline before the advent of chemotherapy (Figs 3.1 and 3.2), probably due to improvement in nutrition and social conditions.

Tuberculosis is caused by *Mycobacterium tuberculosis* (Fig. 3.3); Robert Koch discovered the tubercle bacillus in 1882. The cellular response to tubercle bacilli is the ingestion of the bacilli by macrophages, which are transformed into epithelioid cells. The epithelioid cells fuse to form characteristic giant cells (Langhans' cells). A typical 'tubercle' consists of epithelioid and giant cells surrounded by lymphocytes, the centre of the lesion

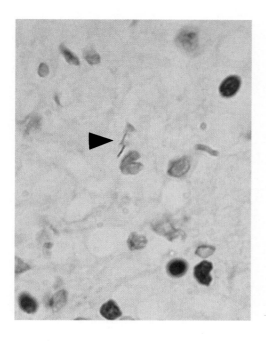

FIGURE 3.3 *Mycobacterium tuberculosis* (arrowed), demonstrated by Ziehl–Neelsen staining.

eventually caseating as delayed hypersensitivity develops (Figs 3.4 and 3.5).

Tuberculous infection may be defined as a state in which the tubercle bacillus is established in the body without symptoms or detectable evidence of disease. Tuberculous disease is a state in which one or more organs of the body become diseased, as shown by bacteriological, radiological or clinical means.

Until recently, most people were infected during some stage of their lives, but many of the younger generations in developed countries have never been infected. In the developing world, however, infection is almost universal. Most people who are infected with the tubercle bacillus, as indicated by a positive Mantoux test, remain well: only 5–15 percent develop tuberculosis. The majority of tuberculous disease is respiratory, but about 10–30 percent is non-respiratory. The incidence of non-respiratory tuberculous disease in the United Kingdom is higher in immigrants from the Asian subcontinent than in British-born Caucasians (Figs 3.6 and 3.7).

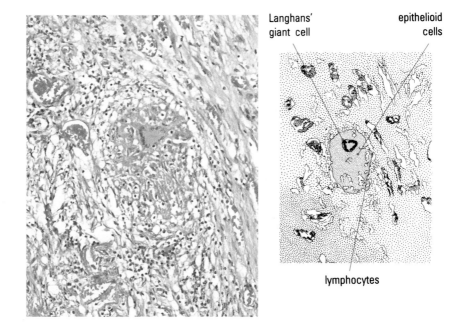

FIGURE 3.4   An early tuberculous follicle or granuloma consisting of epithelioid macrophages, a central Langhans' giant cell and a few peripheral lymphocytes. Haematoxylin and eosin stain.

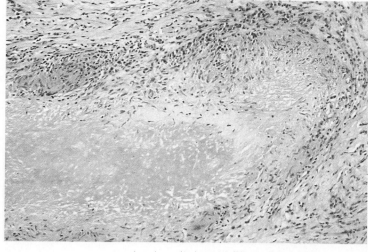

FIGURE 3.5 A caseating epithelioid and giant cell granuloma. Such granulomas are just visible to the naked eye and constitute the 'tubercles' which give the disease its name. Haematoxylin and eosin stain.

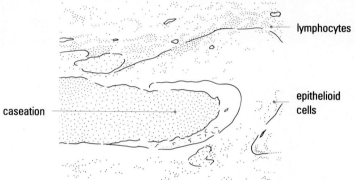

lymphocytes

epithelioid cells

caseation

Incidence of tuberculosis in Caucasians and other ethnic groups			
ethnic origin	overall	respiratory	non-respiratory
Caucasian	9.4	7.9	1.9
Indian	354	237	156
Pakistani and Bangladeshi	353	241	147
West Indian	29.6	21.5	9.3
African	124	92	47
Arab	205	153	74
Chinese	102	74	35
Other	63	48	23
total	16.4	12.7	4.9

FIGURE 3.6 Estimated annual notification rates for tuberculosis per 100 000 population for England by ethnic origin in 1978/9.

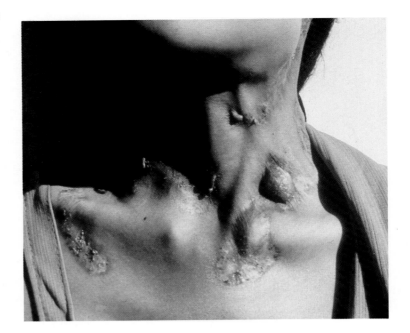

FIGURE 3.7 Enlarged ulcerating cervical lymph nodes due to *Mycobacterium tuberculosis.*

The risk of developing tuberculous disease after infection depends on a number of factors. The young are particularly vulnerable, as are certain ethnic groups, such as Eskimos.

Diabetes, gastrectomy, treatment with immunosuppressive or steroid drugs, and poor nutrition are other predisposing factors. The source of respiratory infection is infected sputum. It is estimated that one patient with positive sputum if untreated, infects ten people per year, or twenty to thirty people before he dies. Each patient is said to cough up 100 million tubercle bacilli per day.

In the United Kingdom, tuberculosis is most commonly found in elderly white males and in immigrants from the Asian subcontinent. In 1980, the annual tuberculosis infection rate for UK children was 0.002 percent; for Indonesia the annual rate was 3–5 percent. Measures that will control the number of cases of tuberculosis are: finding and treating infectious cases; BCG immunization for uninfected individuals; and chemoprophylaxis in certain circumstances.

There are three tuberculin tests in general use: the Mantoux test, the Heaf test and the Tine test. Initial contact with the tubercle bacillus leads to the development of allergy to tubercular protein. This altered state of reaction between the host and the bacillus causes the development of both hypersensitivity and immunity. Hypersensitivity resulting from this infection is cell-mediated, i.e. a type IV reaction (Gell and Coombs). The tuberculin reaction measures the state of tuberculin hypersensitivity of the subject. When tuberculin is injected into the skin of a hypersensitive individual, oedema and hyperaemia occur within a few hours and there is an intensive infiltration of the site with macrophages, polymorphs and lymphocytes. Necrosis may occur in a severe reaction. Such a lesion appears to the naked eye as an area of erythema and induration. This will be visible within 24 hours and will continue to develop for another 48 hours.

PPD is the purified protein derivative of tuberculin; in the United Kingdom a concentrated solution contains 100 000 IU/ml. For many years, when tuberculosis was widespread in the western world, most people reacted to tuberculin and the value of the test was doubtful. However, now that the incidence of tuberculosis is declining in developed countries and most people there do not react to tuberculin, the test has become more useful.

The Mantoux test

The tuberculin used for the Mantoux test is in a series of standard dilutions (Fig. 3.8).

It is advisable to start with the weakest solution of tuberculin in case the patient is strongly hypersensitive. An area of skin on the volar surface of the forearm is cleaned with acetone or ether. A tuberculin syringe and an intradermal needle (Fig. 3.9) are used to inject 0.1ml of tuberculin, strictly intracutaneously (Fig. 3.10). This will produce a wheal 5–8mm in diameter which will disappear within about an hour. If no wheal appears, the tuberculin has been injected too deeply. If the test is positive, an area of erythema and induration will gradually occur after about 24 hours. The test is measured by the diameter of the induration, which is palpated using a finger. The diameter of the induration should be measured in millimetres transversely to the long axis

Standard Mantoux test solutions		
Dilution	Labelled potency	Potency of 0.1ml
1/10 000	10 IU/ml	1 IU
1/1000	100 IU/ml	10 IU
1/100	1000 IU/ml	100 IU

FIGURE 3.8 Standard PPD solutions used in the Mantoux test.

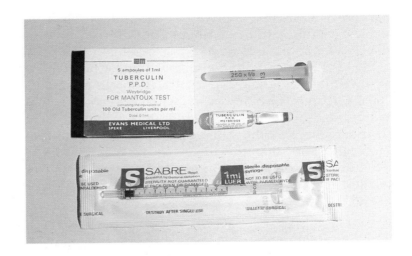

FIGURE 3.9 Mantoux test materials. Courtesy of Dr M. Caplin.

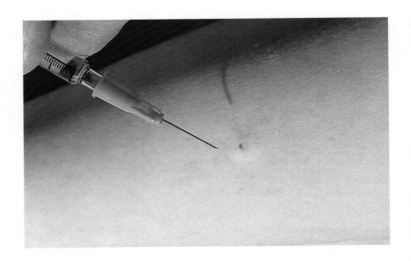

FIGURE 3.10 Intracutaneous Mantoux test producing a wheal of about 5–8mm in diameter. Courtesy of Dr M. Caplin.

of the forearm. In the United Kingdom an induration reaction of 5mm or more is regarded as positive. If the test is negative, then a test using 100 IU can be performed on the other arm. The Mantoux test is the most precise of the tuberculin tests, but it needs skilful injection and is not easy to perform on a wriggling child.

The Heaf test

The Heaf gun (Fig. 3.11) causes six spring-loaded needles to pierce the skin through a drop of undiluted tuberculin. The needle points pierce the skin to a depth of 1–2mm. The gun is sterilized by dipping the endplate and needles into a shallow dish containing methylated spirit and the endplate is then ignited in the flame of a spirit lamp. It is then cooled and the special tuberculin is applied to the dry, clean surface at the junction of the middle and upper third of the volar surface of the left forearm. The skin is then tensed by the operator's left hand and the right hand depresses the handle of the gun, causing the needles to pierce the skin. Any excess tuberculin is removed. A large number of subjects can be tested in a relatively short period using the Heaf gun. Undiluted tuberculin is used, i.e. PPD 100 000 IU/ml, and the resultant reaction is read at 48–72 hours.

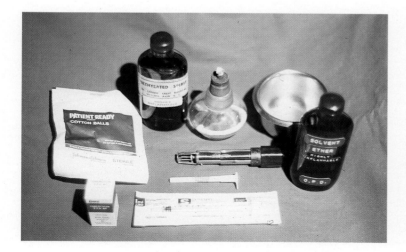

FIGURE 3.11 Heaf test equipment: cotton wool balls, ether for cleaning the arm, methylated spirit and bowl, spirit lamp, needle and syringe, and Heaf gun. Courtesy of Dr M. Caplin.

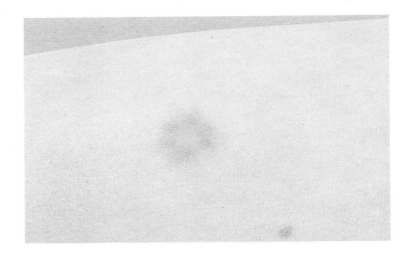

FIGURE 3.12   Heaf Grade I.
Courtesy of Dr M. Caplin.

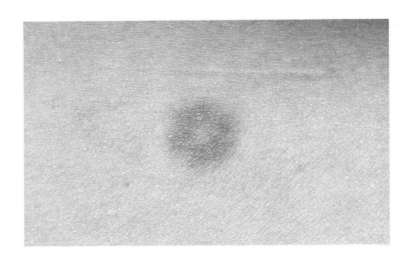

FIGURE 3.13   Heaf Grade II.
Courtesy of Dr M. Caplin.

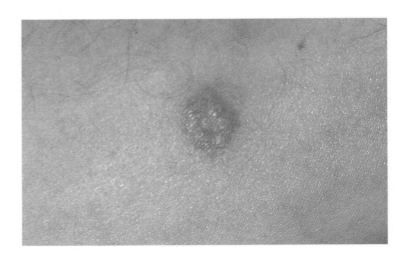

FIGURE 3.14   Heaf Grade IV.
Courtesy of Dr M. Caplin.

The reactions are graded as follows.

Grade I: there is palpable induration around at least four puncture points (Fig. 3.12).

Grade II: the papules are larger and have joined to form a ring (Fig. 3.13).

Grade III: the papules are larger still and have filled in the centre to form a plaque.

Grade IV: the plaque is surmounted by vesicles at the original puncture points and there is surrounding erythema (Fig. 3.14).

The Heaf test is generally considered to be equivalent to about a 10 IU PPD.

The Tine test

This is a disposable multipuncture test (Fig. 3.15). It consists of a plastic holder and baseplate with a stainless steel disc which contains four small tines coated with undiluted tuberculin. The operator tenses the skin with his left hand, and with the right hand firmly applies the tine and presses it onto the skin for 2 seconds. When the unit is lifted there are four visible puncture sites.

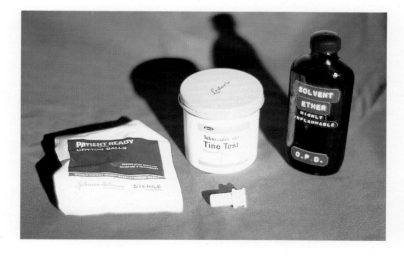

FIGURE 3.15 Tine test equipment. Courtesy of Dr M. Caplin.

The reaction, ranging from Grade I to Grade IV, is read at 48–72 hours.

Grade I: there is palpable induration around at least two puncture points (Fig. 3.16).

Grade II: the papules are larger and just touch; if there are four papules they are joined to form a four-leaved clover shape with a central depression.

Grade III: the papules are larger and have filled in the centre to form a solid plaque.

Grade IV: the plaque is surmounted by vesicles at the original puncture points and there is surrounding erythema (Fig. 3.17).

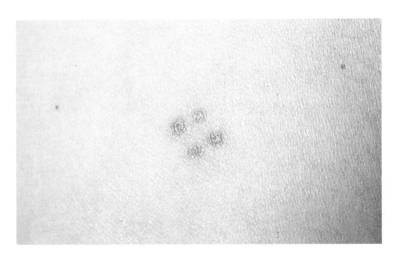

FIGURE 3.16   Tine Grade I.
Courtesy of Dr M. Caplin.

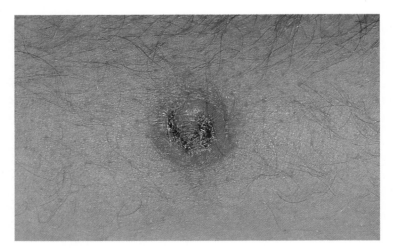

FIGURE 3.17   Tine Grade IV.
Courtesy of Dr M. Caplin.

This test is still relatively expensive, but it is simple to apply and less frightening and painful for children than the Heaf or Mantoux tests. It is essential that the tines are pressed into the skin for the sufficient length of time. The test is weaker than the Heaf test and the standard Mantoux PPD 10 IU test. It is thought to be approximately equivalent to Mantoux 5 IU.

A positive tuberculin reaction may mean that the patient has been infected with tubercle bacilli in the past, has current active tuberculosis or has received BCG vaccination. Tuberculin hypersensitivity may be lost in old age, severe illness of any kind, overwhelming tuberculosis, sarcoidosis, and infectious diseases. It is also often lost during treatment with high doses of corticosteroids.

PRIMARY TUBERCULOSIS

When an individual is infected with the tubercle bacillus for the first time, the tuberculin skin test becomes positive within about three or four weeks. A minority of patients will become pyrexial or develop a hypersensitivity reaction such as erythema nodosum (Figs 3.18 and 3.19), epituberculosis or phlyctenular conjunctivitis. It should be remembered, however, that there are many causes of erythema nodosum other than tuberculosis. In the United Kingdom, for example, the commonest cause is sarcoidosis.

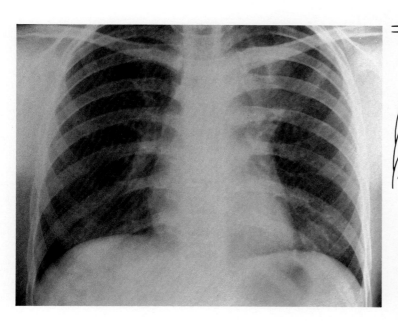

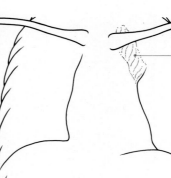

hilar enlargement and partial collapse of left upper lobe

FIGURE 3.18 Chest radiograph of a 12-year-old patient, showing evidence of primary tuberculosis. There is an enlarged left hilar gland and collapse–consolidation, including part of the left upper lobe.

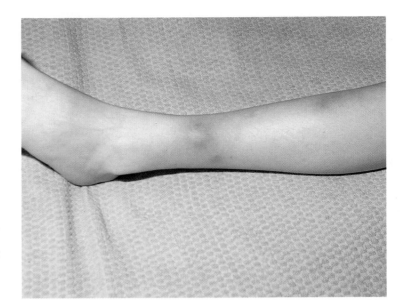

FIGURE 3.19 Erythema nodosum in the same patient as in Fig. 3.18. The contact was her mother who had active pulmonary tuberculosis with positive sputum.

Only about 5–15 percent of people primarily infected with the tubercle bacillus develop overt disease. The radiological appearances of primary tuberculosis include parenchymal involvement, lymphadenopathy, pleural effusions and miliary tuberculosis. The pulmonary lesion is called a Ghon focus (Figs 3.20 and 3.21). In a child, the predominant lesion is an enlarged hilar lymph node (Figs 3.22 and 3.23) with a small peripheral lesion in the lung.

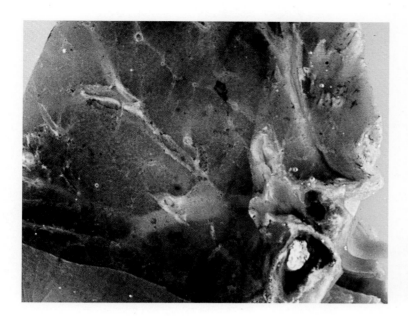

FIGURE 3.20 Gross pathology of a healed primary complex showing the calcified remains of a peripheral Ghon focus and a calcified hilar node.

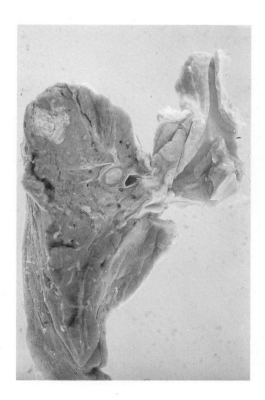

FIGURE 3.21 Primary tuberculous complex in a child, consisting of a peripheral subapical primary lesion (Ghon focus) and massively enlarged hilar lymph nodes, both with extensive caseation.

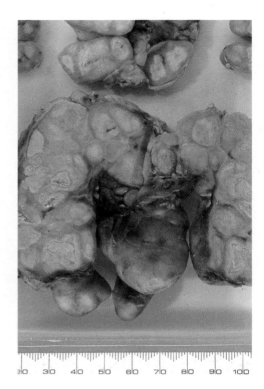

FIGURE 3.22 Mediastinal lymph nodes grossly enlarged and showing confluent areas of caseation.

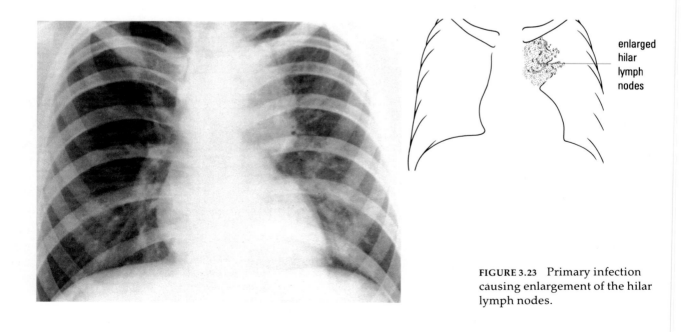

enlarged
hilar
lymph
nodes

FIGURE 3.23 Primary infection causing enlargement of the hilar lymph nodes.

In the majority of patients the primary lesions heal (Figs 3.24 and 3.25). In the adult, the lymph nodes sometimes cause bronchiectasis (Fig. 3.26) or obstructive distension. Bronchial erosion, pleural effusion (Fig. 3.27) and tuberculous bronchopneumonia may occur (Fig. 3.28).

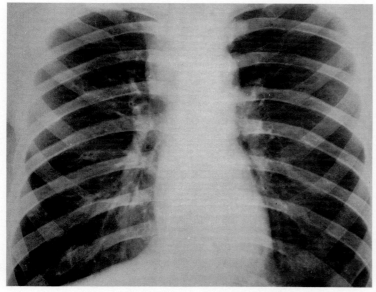

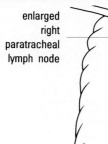

enlarged
right
paratracheal
lymph node

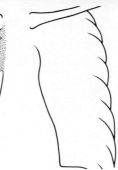

FIGURE 3.24 Enlarged superior mediastinum on the right due to tuberculous adenitis.

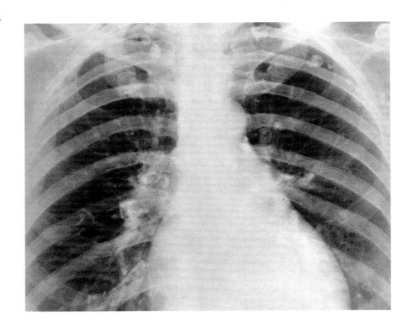

FIGURE 3.25 Widespread calcified nodes in the neck, axilla and mediastinum.

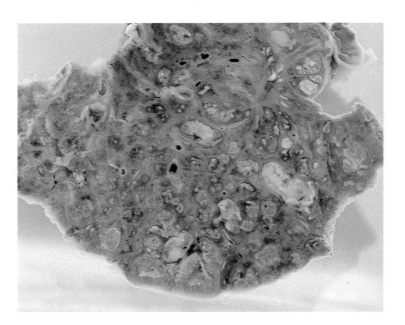

FIGURE 3.26 Tuberculous bronchiectasis.

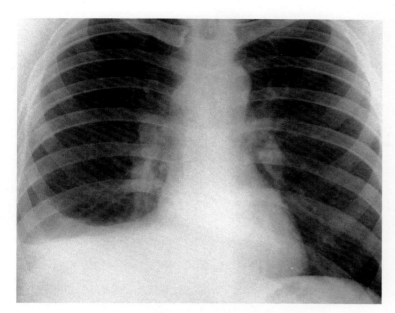

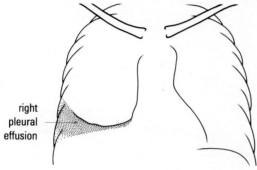

right
pleural
effusion

FIGURE 3.27 Primary
tuberculous pleural effusion.

The most serious complications of primary tuberculosis
are miliary tuberculosis and meningitis.

The diagnosis of primary tuberculosis is by X-ray and
positive skin hypersensitivity to tuberculin. Attempts
should be made to confirm the diagnosis bacteriologic-
ally, but this is often unsuccessful. The treatment is as
for postprimary tuberculosis.

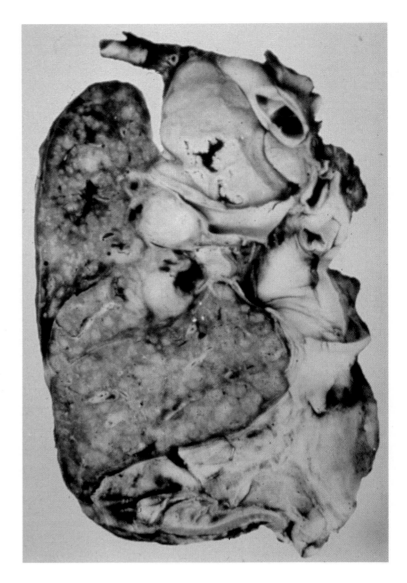

FIGURE 3.28 Tuberculous
bronchopneumonia. Huge
caseating hilar lymph nodes
have ruptured into a major
bronchus, resulting in
widespread caseating
bronchopneumonia.

MILIARY TUBERCULOSIS

Miliary tuberculosis is caused by acute dissemination of the tubercle bacilli via the bloodstream. It usually complicates primary infection in the young (Fig. 3.29). It can, however, occur in a cryptic form in the elderly or immunosuppressed patient. In the acute form in the young person, the patient is acutely ill with a high temperature and cough, but in some cases there are no chest symptoms. The patient may have lymphadeno-pathy and hepatosplenomegaly. The chest X-ray is characteristic, with tubercles of 1.5–3.0mm evenly dist-ributed as nodules throughout both lung fields (Fig. 3.30). The patient may have the classical choroidal tubercles. There are often haematological abnormalities, such as anaemia, leucopenia, thrombocytopenia, pan-cytopenia, leucoerythroblastic anaemia, polycythaemia or disseminated intravascular clotting defects, and there may be electrolyte abnormalities. The diagnosis is by chest radiograph and a positive tuberculin test. Char-acteristic granulomas (Fig. 3.31) and acid-fast bacilli may be found in the marrow, cerebrospinal fluid or in liver biopsy. In some cases of cryptic tuberculosis no granulomas form but many tubercle bacilli can be seen

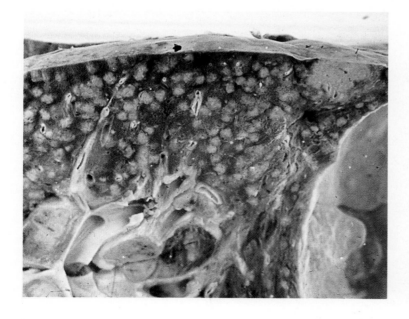

FIGURE 3.29 Primary complex and miliary tuberculosis.

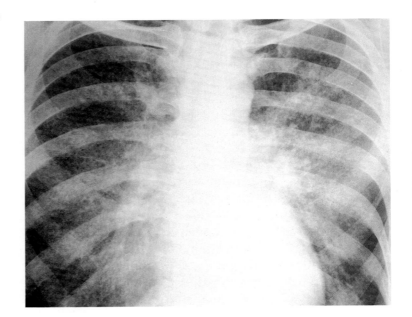

FIGURE 3.30 Miliary tuberculosis. There is widespread fine nodular shadowing in both lungs.

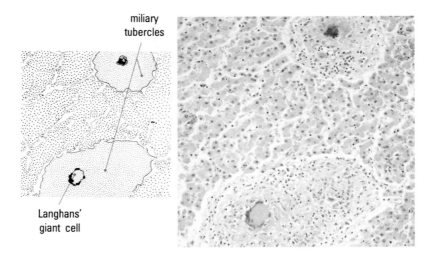

FIGURE 3.31 Miliary tuberculosis. Two miliary tubercles are seen in the liver. Haematoxylin and eosin stain.

with appropriate staining. In the few patients where positive tests cannot be obtained but there is clinical suspicion, a trial of antituberculous drugs should be undertaken. Treatment of miliary tuberculosis is with antituberculous chemotherapy.

Patients with meningitis due to tuberculosis may present with psychological changes, headaches, vomiting and photophobia. Some patients will develop abnormalities of conscious level and focal neurological signs. Severe cases may also benefit from intrathecal steroids and streptomycin.

POSTPRIMARY TUBERCULOSIS

Postprimary tuberculosis can occur as a reactivation of a primary lesion, progression of a primary lesion or, rarely, as a case of reinfection. The patient may present with general symptoms such as weight loss, anorexia, temperature and a general feeling of ill health and/or symptoms specific to the chest such as cough, sputum, dyspnoea, haemoptysis and chest pain. A chest radiograph can reveal a number of appearances, such as pneumonia, particularly in the apical posterior segment of the upper lobe and the apical segment of the lower lobe, fibrosis, cavities, bronchogenic spread, miliary tuberculosis, tuberculomas, pleural effusions and empyema (Figs 3.32–3.39).

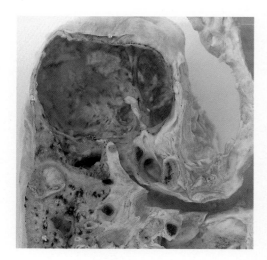

FIGURE 3.32 Postprimary tuberculosis: advanced cavitating apical tuberculosis communicating with the lobar bronchus. The caseous contents have been evacuated and aspiration has led to tuberculous bronchopneumonia in the lower lobe.

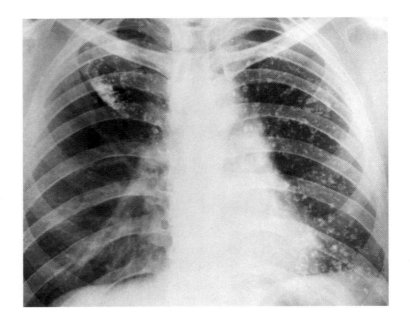

FIGURE 3.33 Postprimary tuberculosis. There is widespread calcification in the left lung and right upper lobe following tuberculous infection.

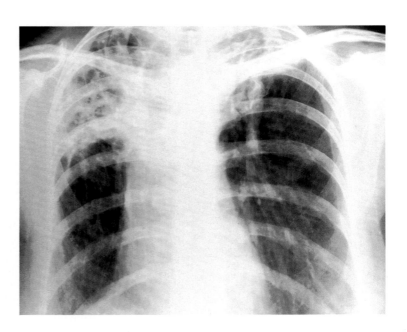

FIGURE 3.34 Postprimary tuberculosis. Severe fibrosis of both upper lobes may be seen.

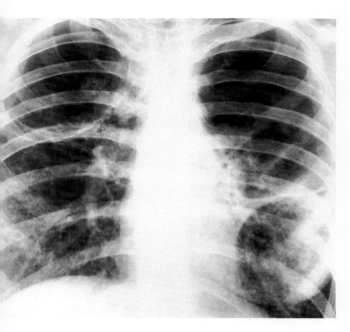
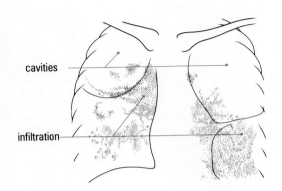

FIGURE 3.35   Postprimary tuberculosis. Tuberculous infiltration of both lungs with thin-walled tension cavities in both upper lobes causes compression of the surrounding lung.

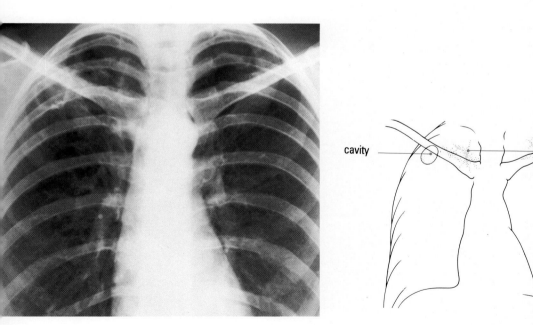
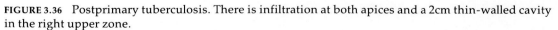

FIGURE 3.36   Postprimary tuberculosis. There is infiltration at both apices and a 2cm thin-walled cavity in the right upper zone.

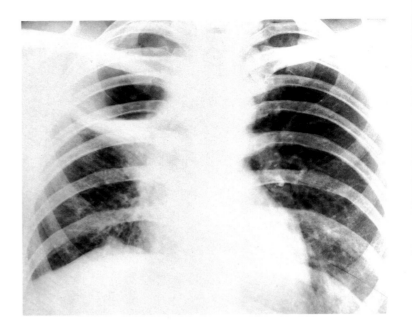

FIGURE 3.37 Postprimary tuberculosis. There is a large cavity with a fluid level in the right upper zone.

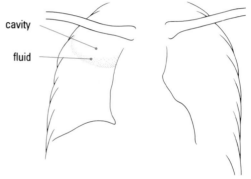

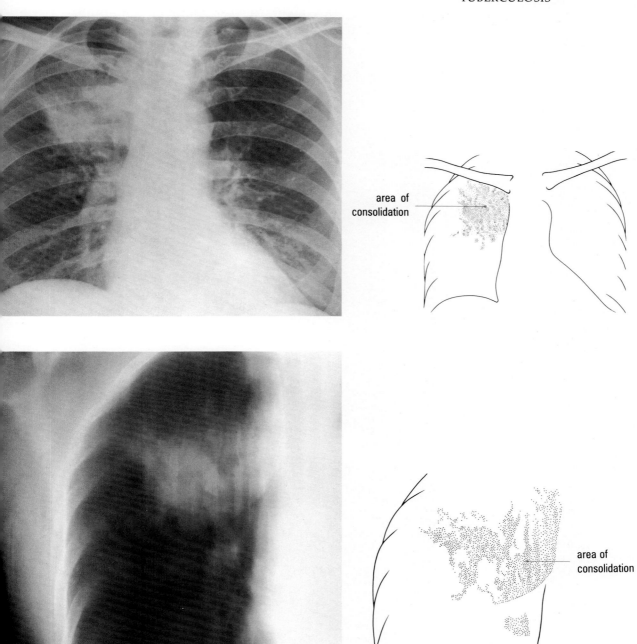

FIGURE 3.38 Postprimary tuberculosis. There is an area of consolidation in the right upper lobe due to tuberculous pneumonia (upper). Tomography of the same patient (lower) shows an air bronchogram.

The diagnosis of postprimary tuberculosis can be confirmed by direct smear of the sputum for acid-fast bacilli, using the Ziehl–Neelsen stain or auramine–rhodamine. If the diagnosis is not confirmed by exami-

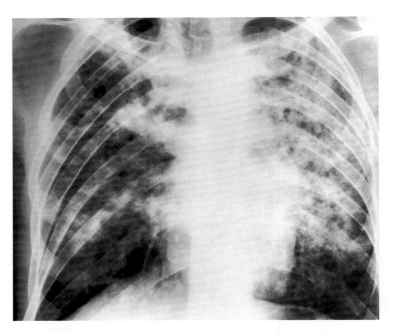

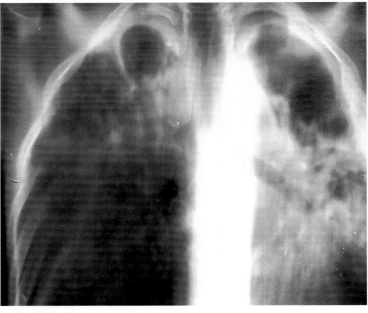

FIGURE 3.39 Postprimary tuberculosis. Severe acute tuberculous infection with cavitation is present (upper). Tomography of the same patient (lower) shows bilateral cavitation.

nation of the sputum, then gastric lavage, laryngeal swabs, biopsy of lymph nodes, and fibreoptic bronchoscopy with washings taken from the bronchial tree may be confirmatory. In a few cases, a trial of antituberculous drugs may be necessary. Effusions should be treated by aspiration and antituberculous drugs; in the case of recurrent effusion, steroids may reduce the amount of residual fibrosis. Empyema can occur; it should be drained and the patient given antituberculous drugs. The patient may be left with residual bronchiectasis, and this may cause recurrent haemoptysis. In some patients, an aspergilloma may develop in an old tuberculous cavity. Other patients have residual tuberculomas (Fig. 3.40) or old, calcified apical lesions (Figs 3.41 and 3.42).

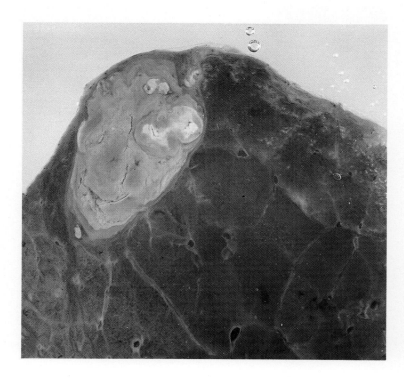

FIGURE 3.40 Postprimary tuberculosis. A tuberculoma represents a quiescent postprimary lesion in the apex of the lung. Although caseous, the edge of the lesion is well demarcated and the lesion is neither progressing nor healed.

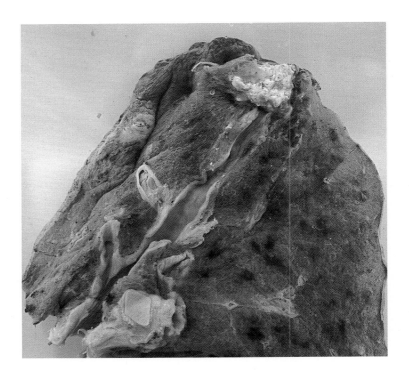

FIGURE 3.41 Postprimary tuberculosis. There is a calcified healed apical lesion.

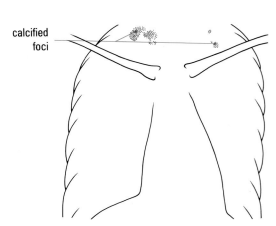

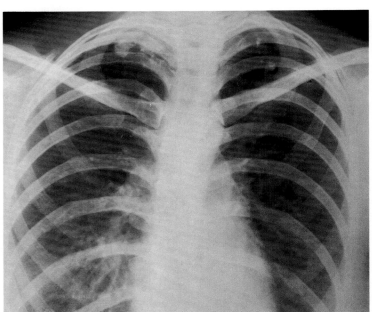

FIGURE 3.42 Postprimary tuberculosis. The chest radiograph shows calcified foci at both apices.

It should be remembered that tuberculosis can affect sites other than the lung. The most common extrapulmonary sites are the lymph nodes. When enlargement of the mediastinal lymph nodes is seen, the differential diagnoses are tuberculosis, sarcoid, lymphoma and carcinoma. Tuberculous ulcers may occur in the skin (Fig. 3.43) and the larynx (Fig. 3.44).

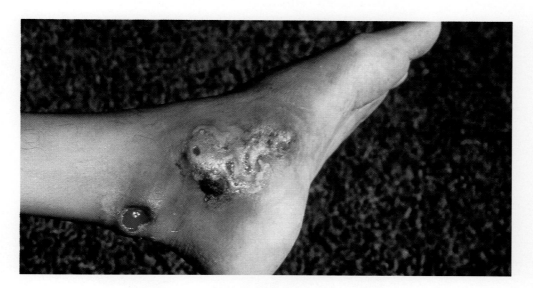

FIGURE 3.43 Ulcers of the foot due to *Mycobacterium tuberculosis*.

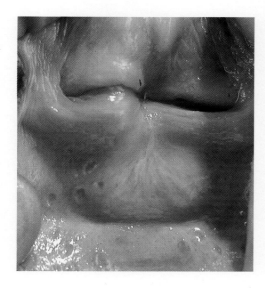

FIGURE 3.44 Tuberculous ulcers of the larynx.

Genitourinary tuberculosis can be serious if it causes a hydronephrosis. A patient with genitourinary tuberculosis requires imaging with ultrasound or intravenous urography at intervals during treatment to ensure that this complication has not developed. Some patients require steroids, others require surgery.

Bone and joint tuberculosis affects the hips, phalanges and spine, and scoliosis and paraplegia may occur. Treatment is by chemotherapy and in some cases surgery. Pericarditis can develop if a mediastinal lymph node ruptures into the pericardium. Tamponade should be treated with aspiration and antituberculous drugs. A constrictive pericarditis may need surgery in addition to antituberculous drugs.

TREATMENT

Today, treatment of pulmonary tuberculosis is by chemotherapy. In the early decades of this century, before the advent of antituberculous therapy, many patients with tuberculosis were treated by collapse therapy. The aim of this therapy was to collapse the affected part of the lung and allow closure of cavities and healing. Various procedures were employed. Air was introduced into the pleural cavity and an artificial

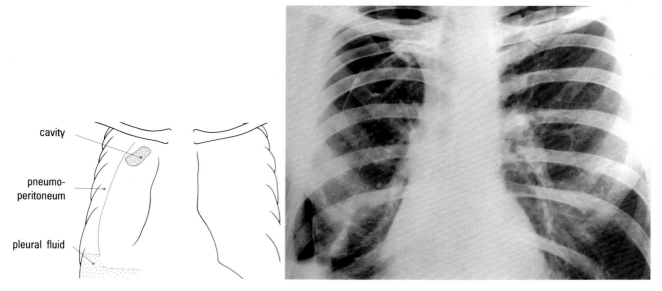

FIGURE 3.45 Artificial pneumothorax on the right, failing to collapse a cavity in the upper part of the right lung. There is also a fluid level at the right base.

pneumothorax was created (Fig. 3.45). The diaphragm was often paralysed by crushing the phrenic nerve in the neck and this treatment was often combined with the introduction of air into the peritoneum — a pneumo-peritoneum (Fig. 3.46). Foreign bodies were introduced extrapleurally — plombage (Fig. 3.47) and many patients had a resection of ribs, allowing the chest wall to cave in — thoracoplasty (Fig. 3.48). These procedures are now of historical interest only but they have been included here because there are still some patients around who owe their lives to these methods of treatment and so these characteristic X-ray appearances will occasionally be seen.

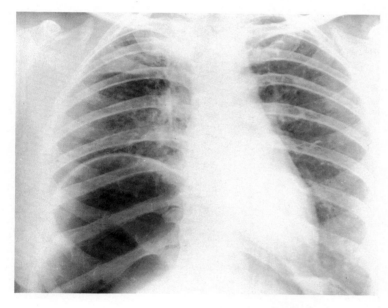

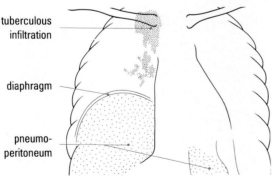

tuberculous infiltration

diaphragm

pneumo-peritoneum

FIGURE 3.46 A right phrenic crush causing paralysis of the right dome of the diaphragm together with a pneumoperitoneum. There is tuberculous infiltration of the right lung, mainly in the upper lobe which is partially collapsed.

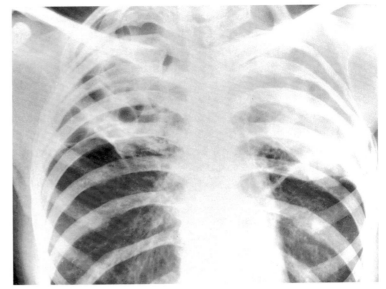

FIGURE 3.47 Bilateral plombage with lucite balls. There are fluid levels in the lucite balls on the right and pressure erosion of the ribs.

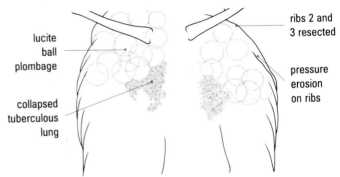

FIGURE 3.48 A seven-rib thoracoplasty causing collapse of the left upper lobe. There are calcified foci in the right upper and middle zones, and scoliosis secondary to the thoracoplasty.

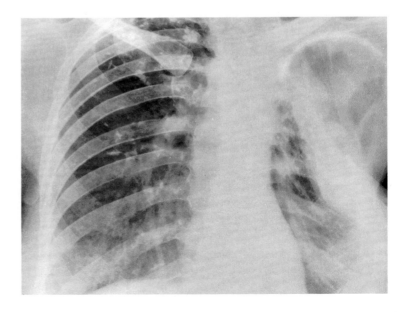

Chemotherapy

Most patients with pulmonary tuberculosis can be managed as outpatients. Once he has started treatment the patient rapidly becomes non-infectious. The indications for hospital treatment are shown in Fig. 3.49.

Primary chemotherapy is the treatment for patients who have never previously had treatment with antituberculous drugs. In the United Kingdom, only about 4 percent of patients have organisms which are resistant to one or more of the main antituberculous drugs. In some of the developing countries the incidence of primary drug resistance is higher. It is to prevent the emergence of drug-resistant organisms that the patients are treated initially with three drugs. The drugs which are suitable for primary chemotherapy are shown in Fig. 3.50.

Para-amino salicylic acid was formerly used as a companion drug with isoniazid and streptomycin, but in developed countries where more effective alternatives can be afforded it is now rarely used.

Treatment is started with three drugs, one of which can be stopped after eight weeks. Treatment is then continued with two drugs. The most commonly used regimen in the United Kingdom is rifampicin, ethambutol and isoniazid for the first two months of treatment, followed by seven months of rifampicin and isoniazid.

Indications for hospital treatment

Severely ill patient

Toxic or allergic reactions to antituberculous drugs

A patient with drug-resistant organisms

An unreliable patient or one with psychiatric or alcohol problems

Adverse social conditions

FIGURE 3.49 Indications for hospital treatment of pulmonary tuberculosis.

Figure 3.51 shows the chest X-rays of a patient before and after treatment with this nine-month regimen. There is evidence that the treatment period can be

Primary therapy for tuberculosis		
Drug	**Dose**	**Details of administration**
streptomycin		intramuscular injection
	1g	daily, if patient <40 years old
	0.75g	daily, if patient >40 years old
	1g	twice weekly with high-dose isoniazid
isoniazid		oral
	300mg	once or twice daily in divided doses
	15mg/kg	twice weekly with streptomycin
thiacetazone		oral
	150mg	single dose daily
ethambutol		oral
	25mg/kg	single dose daily for first 2 months
	15mg/kg	single dose daily, after 2 months
rifampicin		oral
	450–600mg	single daily dose

FIGURE 3.50 Drugs for primary therapy of tuberculosis.

further shortened to six months if, in addition to the treatment described above, pyrazinamide or strepto-mycin is given during the first two months of treatment.

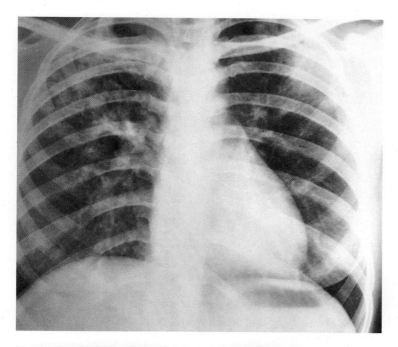

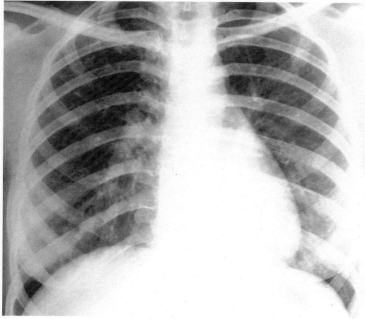

FIGURE 3.51 Before treatment (upper) there is patchy shadowing in both middle and upper zones; after treatment (lower) there is considerable clearing of both lungs.

Supervised intermittent chemotherapy can be used if a patient is unreliable. In this situation, after an initial eight weeks of three drugs the patient can be treated with twice-weekly streptomycin, together with isoniazid. All treatment regimens which do not contain rifampicin should be continued for at least eighteen months.

Retreatment

If a patient has previously taken antituberculous drugs there is a considerable chance that he will have drug-resistant organisms, probably due to inadequate previous therapy. A careful history of previous treatment should be taken and, if possible, the patient isolated and all treatment stopped until the organism has been cultured and its sensitivity assessed. The patient should then be given two drugs to which the organism is fully sensitive. If the organism is still sensitive to them, the drugs listed in Figure 3.50 should be used; if not, more toxic drugs such as ethionamide, prothionamide, pyrazinamide, cycloserine, capreomycin, viomycin or kanamycin must be used. If the patient is so ill that it is not safe to delay the treatment until the sensitivity tests are available, then he should be treated with four or five drugs which he has not previously received.

Adverse reactions to chemotherapy

TOXIC REACTIONS

ISONIAZID.   Peripheral neuropathy can occur; this can be prevented by giving pyridoxine 10mg daily. Psychosis, intellectual impairment, hepatitis, insomnia and epilepsy have also been reported.

ETHAMBUTOL.   A reversible form of optic neuritis which presents as blurring of vision may occur. Red/green colour blindness with a central scotoma may be associated. When a dose of 15mg/kg is used problems are rarely encountered, but patients should be warned to discontinue therapy and report to their doctor if their vision becomes altered in any way. This drug is excreted mainly by the kidneys and is contraindicated in renal insufficiency.

RIFAMPICIN.   Mild gastrointestinal disturbances and impaired liver function may occur. The patient may be alarmed as his sputum and urine become pink and he should be warned that this may happen. A baseline liver function test should be checked before treatment with rifampicin. Most patients have a transient abnormality of their liver function tests about two weeks after commencing treatment with the drug. Rifampicin induces microsomal enzymes and also alters the metabolism of steroids, anticoagulants and oestrogens. A patient taking the contraceptive pill may need to take extra contraceptive precautions during treatment with rifampicin.

STREPTOMYCIN. This can cause vestibular disturbances with nystagmus, ataxia, vertigo or deafness. Nursing staff can develop hypersensitivity to the drug if they are giving frequent injections.

Toxic reactions associated with the drugs used for re-treatment are shown in Figure 3.52.

Drugs for retreatment – toxic reactions	
Capreomycin	nephrotoxicity hypokalaemia ototoxicity
Cycloserine	epilepsy mental disturbance depression
Ethionamide	gastrointestinal upsets
Prothionamide	hepatotoxicity mental disturbance neuropathy
Pyrazinamide	hepatotoxicity hyperuricaemia, gout fever

FIGURE 3.52 Toxic reactions to drugs used for retreatment of tuberculosis.

About 15 percent of patients have allergic reactions to either para-amino salicylic acid or streptomycin. These usually take the form of fever, rash, pruritis or lymphadenopathy. In developed countries, however, para-amino salicylic acid and streptomycin are now used far less frequently than previously. If a patient does develop an allergic reaction, it is best managed by replacing the offending drug. In the past, alternative measures were the use of steroids to suppress the allergic reaction or hyposensitization to the offending drug.

Other aspects of treatment

Follow-up of all patients who have been known to take their drugs conscientiously can be limited to two years from the end of treatment.

Time should be taken to explain to the patient which drugs he must take when and the importance of continuing for the full course of treatment. Patients tend to want to stop treatment when they begin to feel better and this must not be allowed to happen. When they come to clinic, a careful check should be made that they are taking the right drugs in the right dose. If patients are unreliable they should be given supervised chemotherapy.

Close home contacts of a patient who is sputum-positive should be examined and managed as follows. An adult with a positive chest X-ray should be given full antituberculous chemotherapy. An adult with a negative chest X-ray and a negative tuberculin test should be given BCG vaccination. If the tuberculin test is positive he should have a follow-up chest X-ray at six-monthly intervals for two years to make certain he is not developing pulmonary tuberculosis.

A child with a negative radiograph and a negative tuberculin test should be reviewed in six weeks (during which time he should not be in contact with the patient unless the patient is on adequate chemotherapy). If the tuberculin test is still negative at six weeks he should be given BCG. If the radiograph is negative and the tuberculin test positive he should be given isoniazid. If the radiograph is positive he should be given full antituberculous chemotherapy.

Primary chemoprophylaxis is when isoniazid is given to a tuberculin-negative baby because of a smear-positive mother. Isoniazid-resistant BCG is usually given at the same time. Secondary prophylaxis is the more commonly used; this is when a person is infected but without obvious disease. The following may be given secondary chemoprophylaxis: a recent skin test convertor who is a known contact of smear-positive tuberculosis; a child under five years of age with a positive skin test; immigrants, refugees or patients needing to receive immunosuppressive drugs who are known to be Mantoux-positive. Isoniazid is given to adults in a dose of 300mg daily for six months, and to children as 6mg/kg daily for six months.

If a patient has poor renal function the most suitable antituberculous drugs are rifampicin, isoniazid and pyrazinamide, as these are metabolized by the liver. Ethambutol and streptomycin should be avoided.

Pregnant patients should not be given para-amino salicylic acid as the baby may develop a goitre, or streptomycin, which might damage the child's hearing. Rifampicin and ethambutol in high doses have been reported to be teratogenic in animals but have not been reported to cause problems in the human embryo. If a patient who is pregnant needs treatment for her tuberculosis, rifampicin, isoniazid and ethambutol should be satisfactory. By the time the patient realizes that she is pregnant, the most dangerous time (the first twelve weeks) is probably over. Patients who are not pregnant should be advised not to become pregnant whilst taking antituberculous treatment.

Steroids should never be given unless the patient is on adequate antituberculous drugs. However, they may be helpful in a severely ill patient with tuberculous meningitis, in the treatment of allergic reactions to drugs, and in patients with large recurrent tuberculous effusions.

Surgery is indicated only in patients with localized lesions who are unable, or unwilling, to take chemotherapy. Occasionally it is necessary if an old tuberculous cavity becomes colonized with *Aspergillus fumigatus* and an aspergilloma develops. On occasions life-threatening haemoptysis can result and surgery is indicated.

Reasons for treatment failure

The most common reason for failure of treatment is that the patient has taken the drug irregularly. Other reasons for treatment failure are prescription of inadequate drug regimens or the presence of drug-resistant organisms (unusual in the United Kingdom).

Other mycobacteria can cause human pulmonary disease similar to tuberculosis. The organisms most commonly involved are *Mycobacterium kansasii, M. intracellulare, M. avium, M. xenopi* and *M. fortuitum*.

Chapter 4

Viral Chlamydial Rickettsial and Mycoplasmal Pneumonias

VIRAL, CHLAMYDIAL,
RICKETTSIAL
AND MYCOPLASMAL
PNEUMONIAS

Viruses which may cause pneumonia include influenza virus (Figs 4.1 and 4.2), measles virus, cytomegalovirus, adenoviruses, parainfluenza viruses, rhinoviruses, varicella virus, herpes viruses and respiratory syncytial virus.

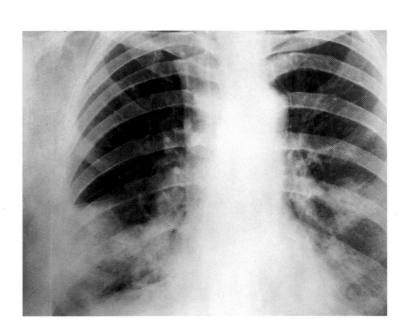

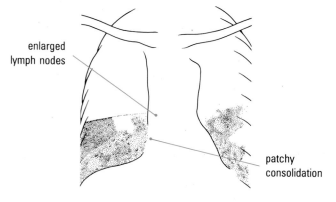

FIGURE 4.1 Influenza virus pneumonia. Non-segmental, poorly defined areas of opacification are present predominantly in the middle lobe and lingula. The patient had a temperature of 39.9°C, a white cell count of $12 \times 10^9/l$ and no response to antibiotics. A complement fixation text revealed a four-fold rising titre to influenza A.

Viral pneumonias are frequently of the interstitial type, with involvement of the alveolar walls and the production of an intra-alveolar exudate. On the chest radiograph there is widespread homogeneous shadowing and there may be an air bronchogram because the airways remain patent and contrast with the consolidation.

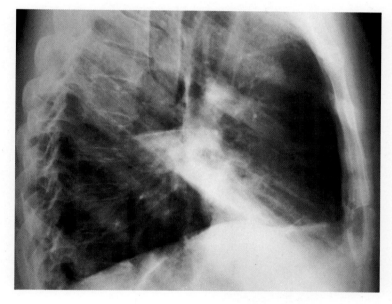

FIGURE 4.2 Influenza virus pneumonia. Lateral view of the patient in Fig. 4.1.

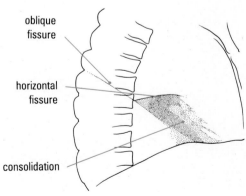

HERPES SIMPLEX VIRUS (HSV)

Among the most common viruses to cause pneumonia in the immunocompromised host are herpes viruses (Fig. 4.3); these have a DNA core and can replicate within the nucleus of infected cells. In normal individuals, HSV produces a localized lesion or 'cold sore', but in immunocompromised patients the sore may spread (Fig. 4.4) and a viraemia may occur, followed by

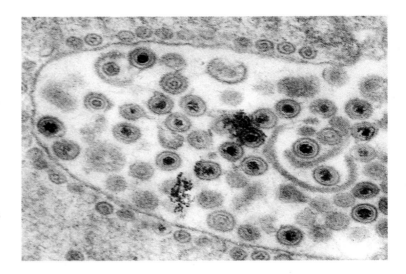

FIGURE 4.3 Herpes simplex virus. Virus particles are ranged along the inside of the cell membrane. Other virus particles have passed through the cell membrane, acquiring an outer envelope.

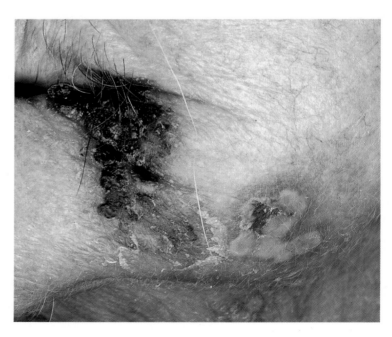

FIGURE 4.4 Herpes simplex virus cutaneous lesion. This spreading lesion occurred in an elderly patient who had received cytotoxic chemotherapy for chronic lymphocytic leukaemia.

the development of pneumonia. In other cases, HSV pneumonia may develop without any preceding cutaneous manifestation (Fig. 4.5). Usually there is a rise in specific antibody titre. Acycloguanosine (acyclovir) intravenously or, in larger doses, orally is the treatment of choice.

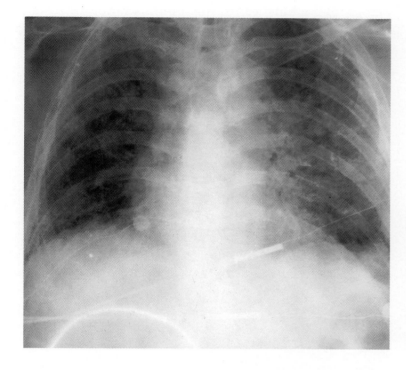

FIGURE 4.5 Herpes simplex virus pneumonia. The chest radiograph of a man aged 55 who had received a high dosage of corticosteroids for cryptogenic fibrosing alveolitis. The bilateral interstitial pneumonia has a rather patchy appearance. HSV was isolated from his sputum.

VARICELLA/ZOSTER VIRUS

Varicella/zoster virus usually manifests itself first as cutaneous, vesiculating lesions which may become haemorrhagic if the patient is thrombocytopenic (Fig. 4.6). This may be followed or accompanied by the development of pneumonia (Fig. 4.7).

The most effective treatment is with intravenous acyclovir; before this was available some benefit was obtained with cytarabine or adenine arabinoside (Ara-A).

If a history of contact with chickenpox is obtained before the rash develops, the administration of zoster immune globulin may reduce the severity of the ensuing infection.

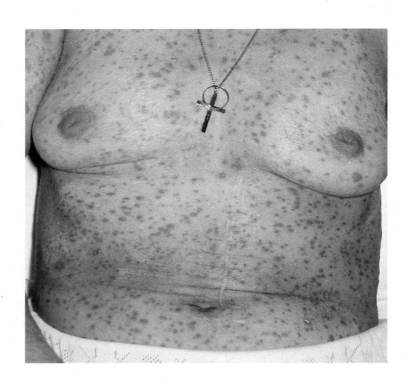

FIGURE 4.6 Varicella/zoster virus cutaneous lesions. This 56-year-old woman was receiving chemotherapy for Hodgkin's disease. Individual lesions had become haemorrhagic because of concurrent thrombocytopenia.

Varicella pneumonia may also complicate severe chickenpox in normal individuals; this is unusual in children but quite frequent in adults, when the pneumonia may develop two to five days after the rash.

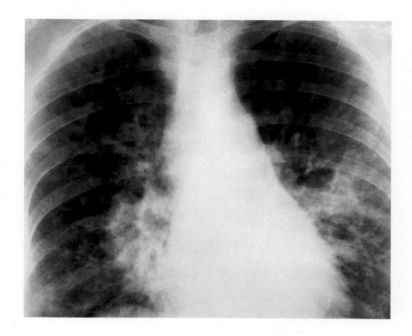

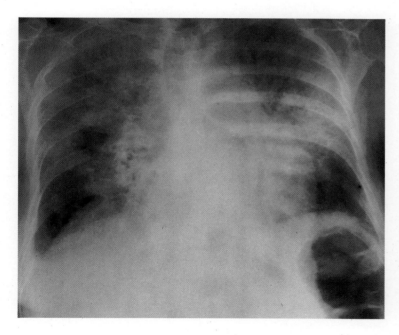

FIGURE 4.7 Varicella/zoster virus pneumonia. The chest radiograph of the patient in Fig. 4.6, taken 24 hours later shows bilateral patchy consolidation (upper). Five days later there was extensive bilateral interstitial shadowing and a marked air bronchogram (lower).

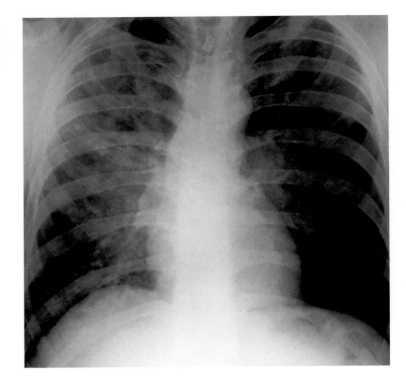

FIGURE 4.8   Varicella/zoster virus pneumonia. This 30-year-old man presented with severe chickenpox. The chest radiograph shows typical confluent nodular infiltrates, mainly in the right mid-zone. After six days of treatment with acyclovir the chest radiograph showed almost complete resolution.

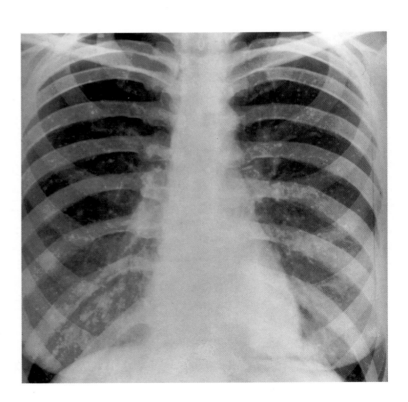

FIGURE 4.9   Varicella/zoster virus pneumonia. This 45-year-old woman had had severe chickenpox ten years previously and her chest radiograph shows typical widespread small healed and calcified lesions.

The chest radiograph shows diffuse small nodular infiltrations (Fig. 4.8) which may eventually leave widespread small calcified nodules (Fig. 4.9).

The histology of chickenpox pneumonia is illustrated in Figure 4.10.

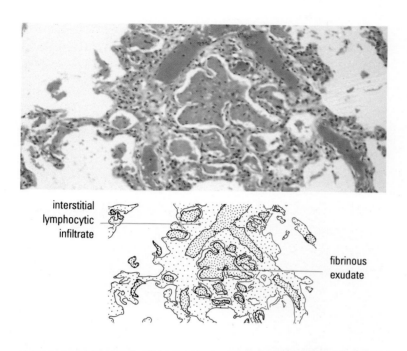

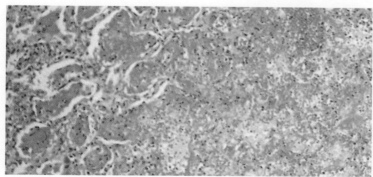

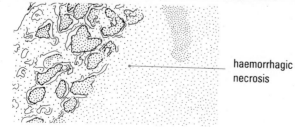

FIGURE 4.10 Chickenpox pneumonia. The early lesion (upper) consists of a small focus of fibrinous exudate surrounded by an interstitial lymphocytic infiltrate. The lesion grows to involve many alveoli (lower) which show haemorrhagic necrosis. Haematoxylin and eosin stain.

CYTOMEGALOVIRUS (CMV)

Cytomegalovirus is a herpesvirus that is transmitted with transfused blood products and will cross the placenta. It causes jaundice, hepatosplenomegaly, haemolysis, mental retardation and pneumonia in neonates, and an illness resembling infectious mononucleosis, with the addition of bronchitis or pneumonia, in adults. Infection in previously healthy individuals may be asymptomatic.

In immunosuppressed patients latent CMV infection may be reactivated or the virus may be acquired from transfused blood products or a transplanted organ.

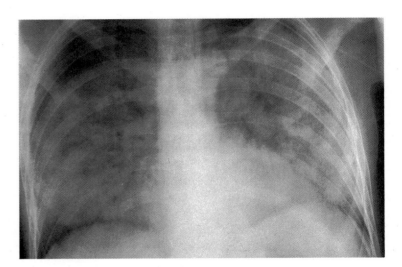

FIGURE 4.11 Cytomegalovirus pneumonia. This 40-year-old man had undergone bone marrow transplantation for acute leukaemia. There is bilateral homogeneous interstitial shadowing with air bronchograms on this radiograph three weeks after the transplant.

The most susceptible patients are those who require frequent blood, platelet or white cell transfusions (for example, bone marrow transplant recipients). There is typically a latent period of 20–40 days before the pneumonia develops, and it is frequently accompanied by hepatitis and by the appearance of abnormal mononuclear cells in the peripheral blood.

Radiographic appearances are similar to those of other viral pneumonias (Fig. 4.11). The diagnosis may be made by observing a significant rise in specific antibody titre or by biopsy of the lung or other affected organs, when the typical 'owl's eye' intranuclear inclusion bodies may be seen (Fig. 4.12). A direct fluorescent antibody test is now available.

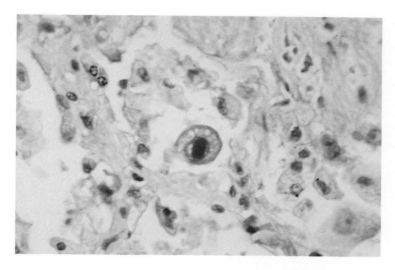

FIGURE 4.12 Cytomegalovirus 'owl's eye' inclusion body. Infected cells increase in size, and large numbers of virus particles accumulate within the nucleus to produce a single dense inclusion. The space between the inclusion and the nuclear membrane, together with the surrounding rim of cytoplasm, give rise to the typical 'owl's eye' appearance. Haematoxylin and eosin stain.

Ganciclovir intravenously is the treatment of choice, and trisodium phosphonoformate (foscarnet) has been used in resistant cases. If pneumonia becomes life-threatening, some advocate high-dosage corticosteroids, with assisted ventilation if required, in the hope of reducing the inflammatory response to the virus and thus the severity of the illness. If the patient's ventilation can be supported, recovery may occur. Some believe that the use of CMV-hyperimmune globulin may reduce the severity of the illness and it improves the response rate to ganciclovir in patients with AIDS. In transplant patients, prevention, by using CMV-negative blood products and transplant donors whenever possible, is the most successful approach.

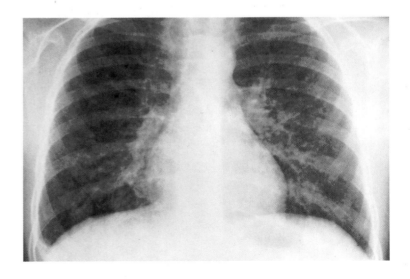

FIGURE 4.13 Measles pneumonia. This radiograph of a 4-year-old boy with acute lymphoblastic leukaemia shows poorly defined patchy shadowing throughout both lungs with an air bronchogram in the left upper zone.

The measles virus sometimes causes interstitial pneumonia (Fig. 4.13) in immunosuppressed children who have not had measles previously or who have not maintained adequate anti-measles virus antibody titres as a result of their immunosuppression. There is usually a history of exposure to measles, and a rash suggestive of measles is usually present. The diagnosis may be confirmed by direct immunofluorescence of nasal swabs which contain the virus particles, or characteristic multinucleate giant cells may be seen in a lung biopsy specimen (Fig. 4.14).

Treatment is unsatisfactory, although some successes have been achieved using interferon with mechanical ventilatory support as required. Measles vaccine should be given to children with leukaemia who do not have detectable antibody in their serum at the start of treatment.

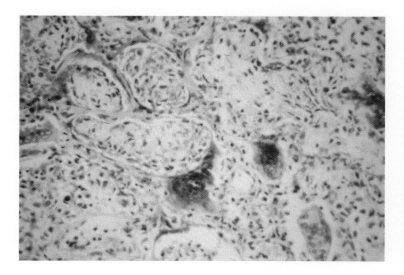

FIGURE 4.14 Measles pneumonia. This lung biopsy specimen shows an inflammatory cell infiltrate and proliferation of the alveolar lining cells. Large, darkly staining, multinucleate giant cells typical of measles pneumonia are present. Haematoxylin and eosin stain.

CHLAMYDIAL, RICKETTSIAL AND MYCOPLASMAL PNEUMONIAS

Pneumonia due to *Chlamydia psittaci* (Fig. 4.15) is usually found where there is a history of contact with birds, and rickettsial pneumonias where there is contact with animals.

Mycoplasmal pneumonia (Figs 4.16 and 4.17) is commonly the cause of outbreaks in schools, military camps and other institutions.

Pneumonia due to viruses, rickettsia, mycoplasma and chlamydia is less dramatic in onset than bacterial pneumonia. There is usually a history of lethargy, fever,

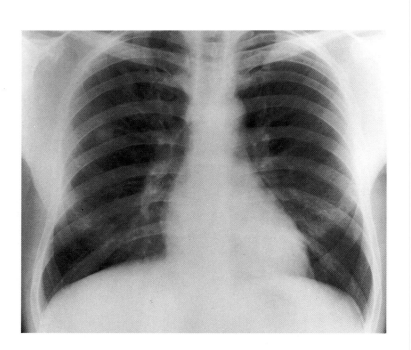

FIGURE 4.15 Psittacosis pneumonia. There are small areas of consolidation in the right upper and mid zones.

headaches and arthralgia before the onset of respiratory symptoms. The white cell count may be normal or low and there may be an increased proportion of lymphocytes. Some patients have few abnormal physical signs in the chest and the radiograph often shows less extensive consolidation than in bacterial pneumonia. Occasional cases may, however, be fulminating.

Chlamydia, rickettsial and mycoplasmal pneumonias benefit from treatment with tetracycline or erythromycin.

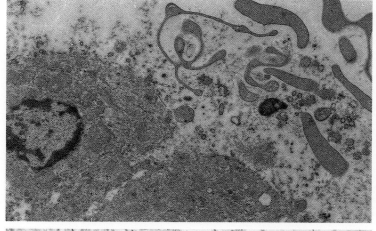
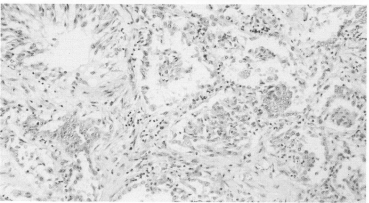

FIGURE 4.16 Mycoplasma pneumonia. The electronmicrograph (upper) shows irregular mycoplasmal organisms on the surface of a degenerate respiratory epithelium. The infected lung section shows proliferating regeneration of the bronchiolar and alveolar epithelium, macrophages in the alveoli and a lymphocytic interstitial infiltrate. Haematoxylin and eosin stain.

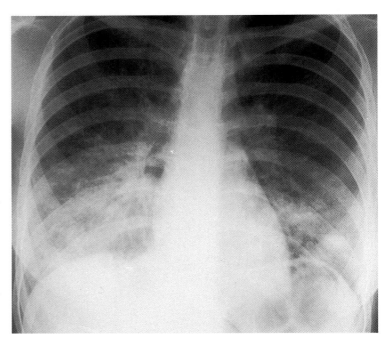

FIGURE 4.17 Mycoplasma pneumonia. This patient presented with eight days of fever, malaise, cough and sputum. The temperature was 39°C and the white cell count 7.5×10^9/l. Cold agglutination and the complement fixation test were positive for *Mycoplasma pneumoniae*.

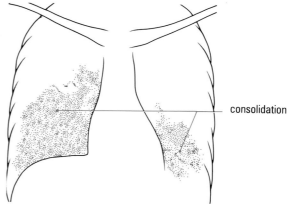

Chapter **5**

Infection by Actinomycetes Fungi and Protozoa

ACTINOMYCETACEAE

This family includes two genera of higher bacteria that may cause disease in man: *Actinomyces* and *Nocardia*. Both occur as Gram-positive rods which branch and form filaments (Fig. 5.1); actinomyces also occur in a fungal form. In *A. israelii*, the fungal form produces characteristic yellow 'sulphur granules' which are usually found in fluid from an empyema or abscess. The organisms are acid alcohol-fast and usually stain with the Ziehl–Neelsen method (Fig. 5.2).

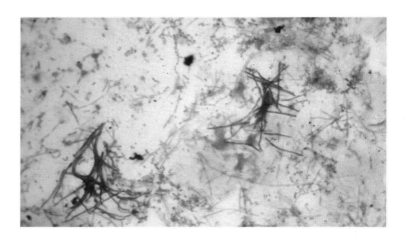

FIGURE 5.1 *Nocardia asteroides.* In the filamentous form both nocardia and actinomyces are Gram-positive, acid alcohol-fast, branching rods and cannot be distinguished morphologically. Ziehl–Neelsen stain.

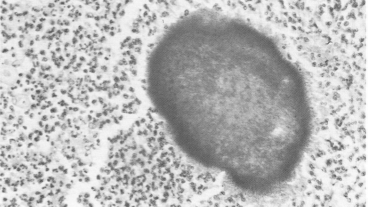

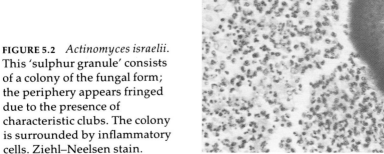

FIGURE 5.2 *Actinomyces israelii.* This 'sulphur granule' consists of a colony of the fungal form; the periphery appears fringed due to the presence of characteristic clubs. The colony is surrounded by inflammatory cells. Ziehl–Neelsen stain.

Actinomyces israelii

Actinomyces israelii is an anaerobic or microaerophilic mouth organism that is usually saprophytic. It may become locally pathogenic or may involve the lungs or gastrointestinal tract by aspiration or by swallowing. In the lungs, actinomycosis is often initially unilateral, taking the form of pneumonia, lung abscess or sinus (Fig. 5.3). Treatment is with benzylpenicillin in high dosage

Nocardia species

Nocardia species are aerobic actinomycetes found in the soil. Lung disease due to nocardia may occur in agricultural workers and in individuals who are immunosuppressed.

Infection characteristically produces multiple nodular opacities on the chest radiograph, and medium-sized and large nodules tend to cavitate (Figs 5.4 and 5.5). A pleural effusion may occur, and there may also be a periosteal reaction with new bone formation at the surface of a rib or vertebra adjacent to a peripheral pulmonary lesion. In immunosuppressed patients, the infection may spread to involve a lobe or a whole lung (Fig. 5.6).

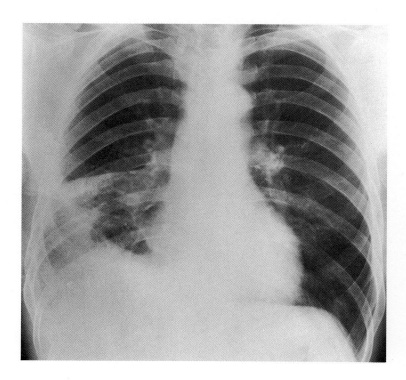

FIGURE 5.3 Actinomycosis. This chest radiograph of a 55-year-old man who had recurrent episodes of right-sided pleuritic chest pain shows consolidation in the periphery of the right middle lobe. *Actinomyces israelii* was isolated from the sputum and the patient responded to benzylpenicillin, 10 megaunits daily.

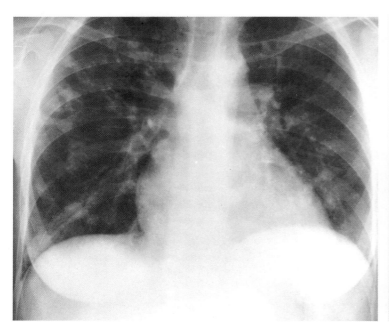
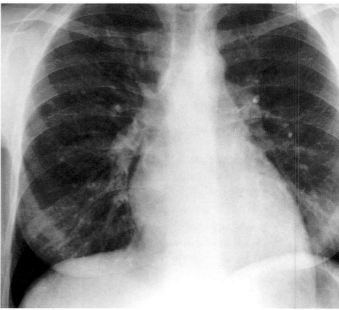

FIGURE 5.4 Pneumonia due to *Nocardia asteroides*. This patient had had a successful renal transplant. Moderately well-defined opacities, 1–2cm in diameter, occur in both lungs (left). Some of the lesions have cavitated and appear as ring shadows. The opacities have almost disappeared after treatment (right).

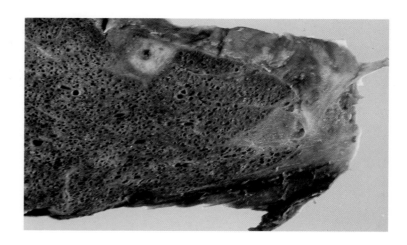

FIGURE 5.5 Nocardiosis. This cut surface of a lung, postmortem, shows two peripheral cavitating nodules and inflammation of the pleura with fibrin deposition.

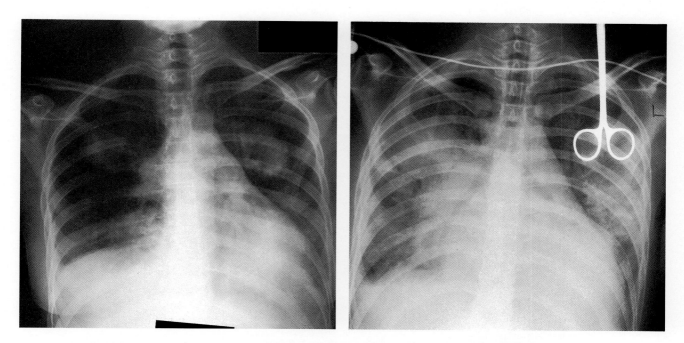

FIGURE 5.6 Nocardiosis. This 31-year-old woman was receiving corticosteroids for systemic lupus erythematosus. She had large round bilateral shadows (left) and forty-eight hours later consolidation had spread throughout both lungs (right).

Sulphonamides are the treatment of choice for most nocardia infections, but for *N. asteroides* there is synergism between co-trimoxazole and erythromycin.

MUCORMYCOSIS

The order Mucorales includes the genera *Mucor*, *Rhizopus* and *Absidia*. These fungi are normally saprophytic but may become pathogenic in immunocompromised individuals (Fig. 5.7). Among cases of fungal pneumonia in such individuals, mucorales are found infrequently; they may be identified to some degree by their morphology (Fig. 5.8), but speciation requires culture. Infection with mucorales responds to intravenous amphotericin B.

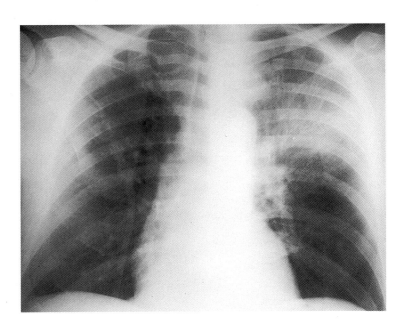

FIGURE 5.7 Mucor pneumonia. This 54-year-old man had received intensive chemotherapy for acute myeloid leukaemia. He complained of cough, breathlessness and pleuritic pain in the left upper chest. The radiograph shows extensive consolidation of the left upper lobe. He was treated for a bacterial pneumonia and the correct diagnosis was only made postmortem.

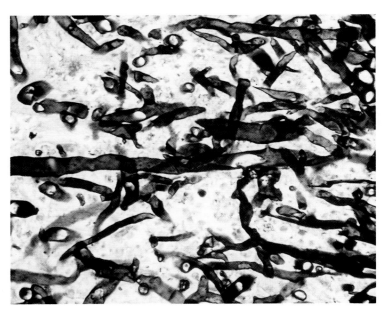

FIGURE 5.8 This lung section from the patient in Fig. 5.7 shows large non-septate hyphae with irregular lateral branching, typical of the Mucorales. Grocott stain.

In immunocompromised individuals, and particularly in patients with diabetes mellitus, a characteristic rhino-cerebral form of mucormycosis infection may occur. From the hard palate the infection typically extends upwards through the maxillary sinus and the floor of the skull to invade the base of the brain (Fig. 5.9). Treatment is by local resection and systemic ampho-tericin B.

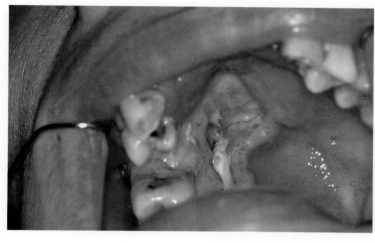

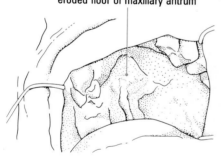

eroded floor of maxillary antrum

FIGURE 5.9 Rhinocerebral mucormycosis. The perforated hard palate of a 26-year-old woman who presented with pulmonary tuberculosis and uncontrolled diabetes mellitus. She wore an upper denture and this lesion was asymptomatic. Sections of the resected lesion showed hyphae typical of the Mucorales.

DISEASES ASSOCIATED WITH *ASPERGILLUS*

Fungi of the genus *Aspergillus* form true hyphae which are septate and show dichotomous branching (Fig. 5.10 left); asexual spores known as conidia are borne on specialized hyphae termed conidiophores (Fig. 5.10 right).

Allergic bronchopulmonary aspergillosis

The spores of *Aspergillus* species are widely distributed in the air and may cause a hypersensitivity reaction when they are inhaled. This reaction may be of the immediate type (Type I), which may produce an attack of allergic asthma, or it may be of Type III, in which intense local inflammation develops in the bronchiolar wall as a result of the reaction between the spores and circulating antibody. The two types of hypersensitivity may coexist, but an episode of allergic bronchopulmonary aspergillosis (ABPA) can sometimes be differentiated from asthma, since in ABPA cough and chest discomfort are often more prominent symptoms than wheezing.

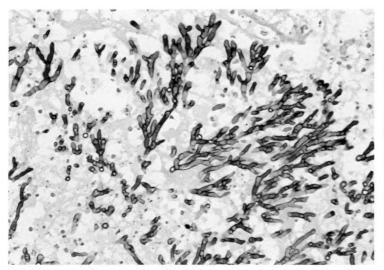 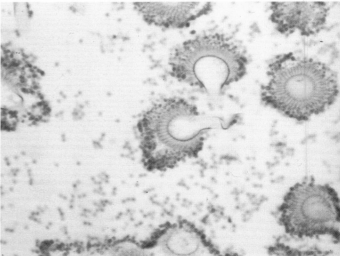

FIGURE 5.10 *Aspergillus* species. The hyphae are septate with regular dichotomous branching (left). Grocott stain. Conidia are borne on conidiophores, shown here in transverse and longitudinal section (right).

The inflammatory reaction of ABPA can result in the formation of a mucus plug (Fig. 5.11). The mucus plug may contain hyphae, and can cause collapse of the segment or lobe distally (Fig. 5.12). When ABPA affects

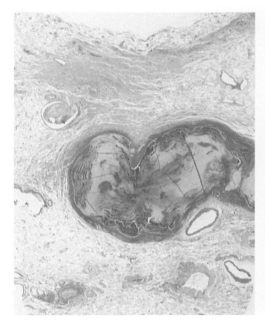
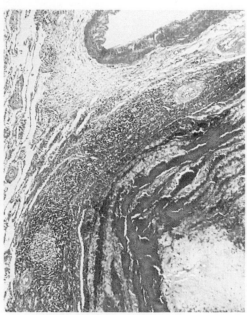

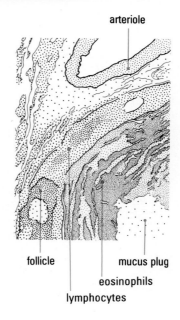

FIGURE 5.11 Allergic bronchopulmonary aspergillosis. A mucus plug containing eosinophilis entirely occludes the lumen of a small bronchus. At higher power large numbers of lymphocytes and a lymphoid follicle are seen in the bronchial submucosa. Haematoxylin and eosin stain.

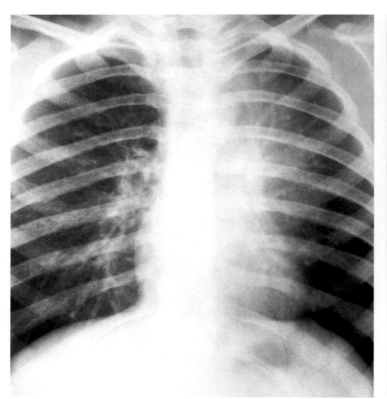 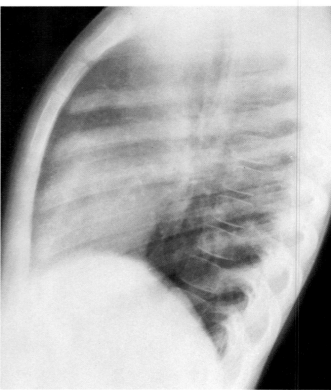

FIGURE 5.12 Bronchopulmonary aspergillosis. This child presented with fever, but without a history of asthma, and a collapsed left upper lobe. A blood eosinophilia and a positive skin prick test to *Aspergillus fumigatus* suggested the diagnosis, and she responded to treatment with corticosteroids. Bronchoscopy showed a mucus plug impacted in the left upper lobe bronchus. The lateral chest radiograph clearly shows left upper lobe collapse.

smaller airways, a number of infiltrates are seen in the lung fields, without collapse, which disappear either spontaneously or following treatment (Fig. 5.13).

ABPA may be diagnosed if there are transient opacities on the chest radiograph, eosinophilia in the blood or sputum, evidence of Type I hypersensitivity to *Aspergillus* species and precipitating antibodies in the serum or a delayed (Type III) reaction to intradermal challenge with aspergillus protein.

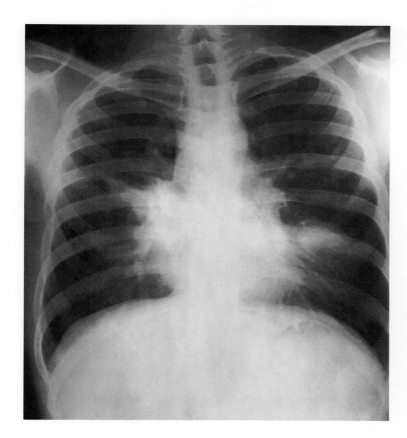

FIGURE 5.13 Allergic bronchopulmonary aspergillosis: transient opacities. The patient had episodic cough and wheeze and a marked blood eosinophilia. There are typical infiltrates in both mid-zones, which cleared rapidly with corticosteroid treatment.

Episodes should be treated with corticosteroids and treatment should be started promptly in order to avoid permanent damage to the bronchial or bronchiolar wall. Repeated attacks without prompt treatment will lead to bronchiectasis, typically of the saccular type in the minor bronchi (Fig. 5.14), and to widespread fibrosis (Fig. 5.15).

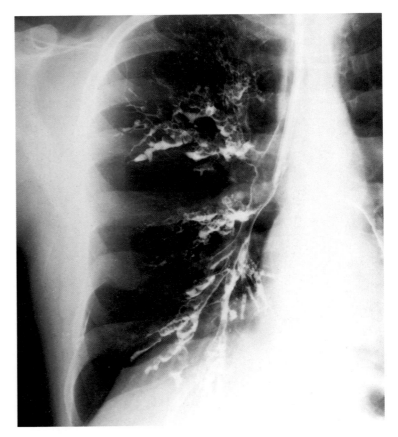

FIGURE 5.14 Bronchopulmonary aspergillosis. Bronchogram showing proximal bronchiectasis with normal peripheral bronchi.

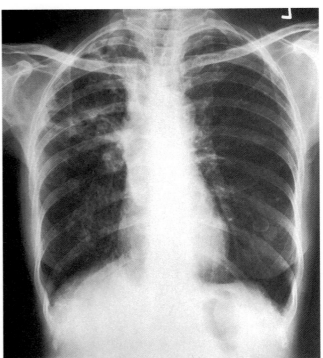

FIGURE 5.15 Allergic bronchopulmonary aspergillosis: fibrosis. Repeated episodes of allergic aspergillosis have caused fibrosis and contraction of the right upper lobe in this 65-year-old woman.

Aspergilloma

When cavitation or extensive fibrous scarring occurs in a lung the site may become colonized by *Aspergillus* species. The resulting fungus ball is termed an aspergilloma (Fig. 5.16). The fungus ball may be expectorated piecemeal, leaving an apparently empty cavity, but active fungal growth in the wall of the cavity will cause the aspergilloma to re-form. Continued increase in the size of the cavity leads to progressive deterioration of lung function. Haemoptysis is frequent and may be massive or even fatal, and high titres of precipitating antibodies are found in the serum.

Treatment with antifungal agents is not successful and therefore surgical removal of the fungus ball and the lobe or segment containing it is the treatment of choice, provided that the remaining lung function is adequate (Fig. 5.17).

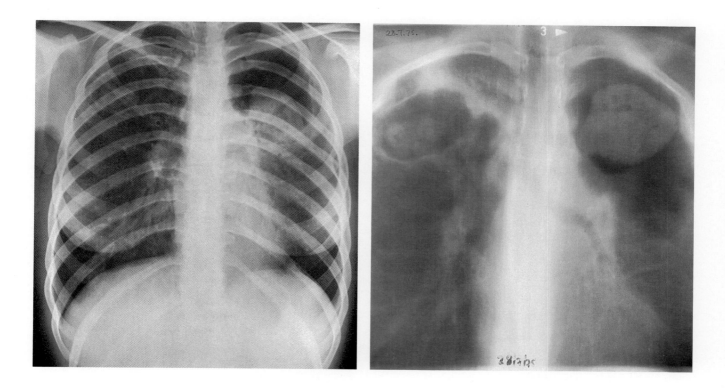

FIGURE 5.16 Aspergilloma. The chest radiograph shows a well-defined cavity containing a fungus ball in the left upper lobe and the same features, less clearly defined, in the right upper lobe. Both aspergillomata are confirmed by the tomogram.

fungal mass

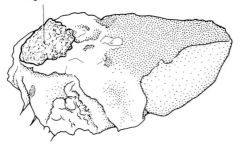

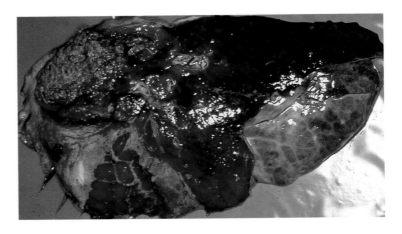

FIGURE 5.17 Aspergilloma: right upper lobectomy specimen. A large mass of fungus is present within a fibrotic cavity in the apex.

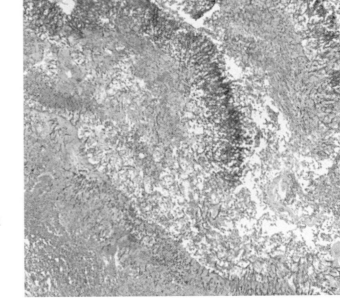

FIGURE 5.18 Invasive aspergillosis. The bronchial lumen contains several masses of aspergillus, and the bronchial wall has been invaded by hyphae. A brisk inflammatory response is present in the submucosa. Haematoxylin and eosin stain.

Invasive aspergillosis

In immunocompromised individuals *Aspergillus* species may not remain confined within a bronchus or cavity, but may rapidly progress into the lung parenchyma (Fig. 5.18). If cavitation or prior lung damage has occurred for any reason, colonization and invasion may be extremely rapid, especially if the patient is severely neutropenic (Fig. 5.19).

Aspergillus pneumonia may produce a variety of appearances on the chest radiograph, including multiple nodules which may cavitate (Fig. 5.20) and widespread reticular shadowing (Fig. 5.21).

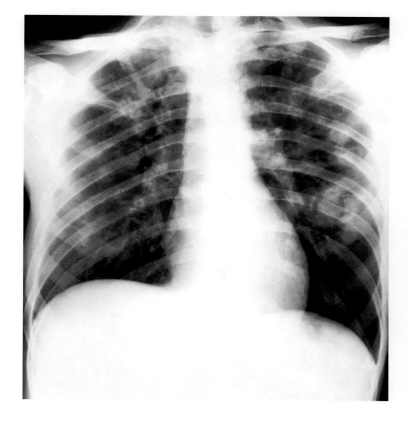

FIGURE 5.19 Invasive aspergillosis. This chest radiograph of a man with acute myeloid leukaemia, who developed a *Staphylococcus epidermidis* bacteraemia from a central venous catheter, shows numerous small cavities in the lung fields. A cavity at the right apex and one in the left mid-zone have become opacified because of secondary colonization with *Aspergillus fumigatus*.

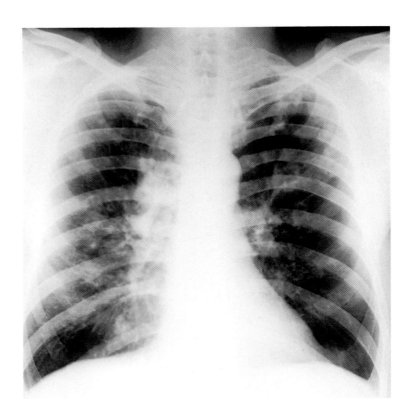

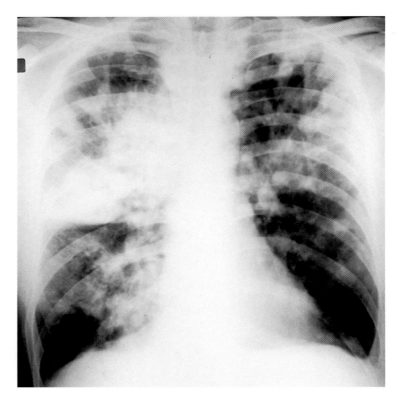

FIGURE 5.20 Aspergillus pneumonia. Chest radiograph of a patient with very severe asthma, only controlled by prednisolone 120mg daily; on this regimen he developed increasing breathlessness and bilateral widespread shadows (upper). His sputum contained *Aspergillus fumigatus* and no other pathogen. One week later, there was rapid extension of shadowing (lower) despite intravenous amphotericin B and attempted lowering of prednisolone dosage. Autopsy showed extensive invasive aspergillosis.

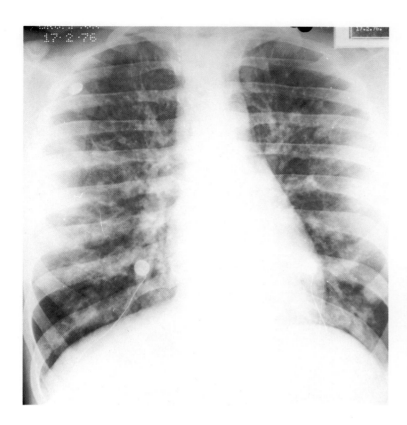

FIGURE 5.21 Aspergillus pneumonia. Widespread patchy shadowing with small cavities is present throughout both lung fields. The patient was a 21-year-old woman who had required mechanical ventilation and a high dosage of corticosteroids for severe status asthmaticus.

Aspergillus species have a predilection for invading pulmonary arterioles and venules (Fig. 5.22). This may result in pulmonary infarction accompanied by pleuritic chest pain, and early dissemination of the fungus via the blood. Since the lungs provide the usual portal of entry for *Aspergillus* species they are almost always involved in disseminated aspergillosis (compare candidosis), but the brain is the second commonest site of involvement (Fig. 5.23).

Aspergillus pneumonia and disseminated aspergillosis should be treated with intravenous amphotericin B together with 5-fluorocytosine, but the outcome depends upon successful reversal of immunosuppression and, particularly, upon the reversal of neutropenia.

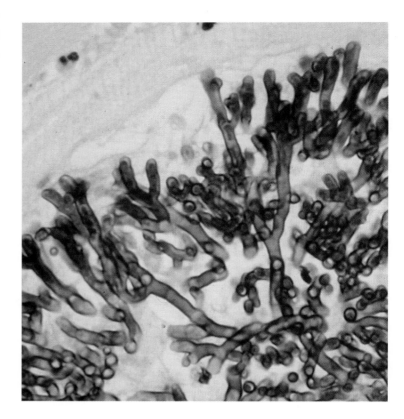

FIGURE 5.22 Invasive aspergillosis. Hyphae are growing within the lumen of an arteriole in this postmortem specimen from a patient with chronic airways obstruction who had required mechanical ventilation, broad-spectrum antibacterial therapy and corticosteroids. Grocott stain.

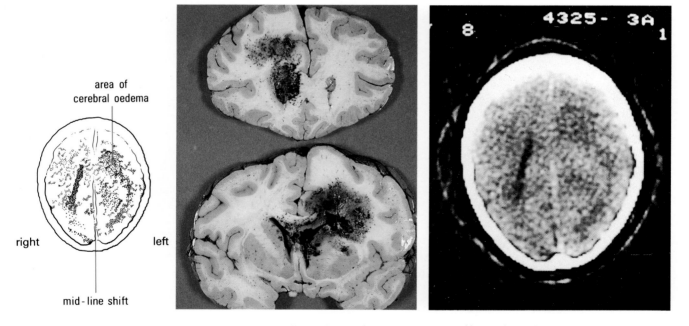

area of
cerebral oedema

right   left

mid-line shift

FIGURE 5.23 Disseminated aspergillosis: brain abscess. A section of brain from the patient in Fig. 5.21 shows haemorrhagic necrosis extending from the left lateral ventricle into the white matter of the parietal lobe. There is also considerable swelling of the left side of the brain. The CT scan shows little change in density of the affected brain substance on the left, but cerebral oedema is marked.

CANDIDOSIS (MONILIASIS)

Patients who are seriously ill, debilitated or immuno-suppressed may experience increased colonization of the mouth and pharynx by *Candida* species, most commonly *Candida albicans*. This organism is a normal commensal of mucous membranes but frequently becomes locally invasive, causing oral candidosis (Fig. 5.24).

Since *C. albicans* is present in the oropharynx of most normal individuals, great care has to be taken that secretions expectorated from the lower respiratory tract do not become contaminated and thus lead to an erroneous diagnosis of candida pneumonia.

Severe oral candidosis is frequently accompanied by candida oesophagitis (Fig. 5.25) which causes retrosternal discomfort or pain, aggravated by swallowing. When candida oesophagitis develops it is frequently followed by deep invasion and systemic spread of the organism via the bloodstream.

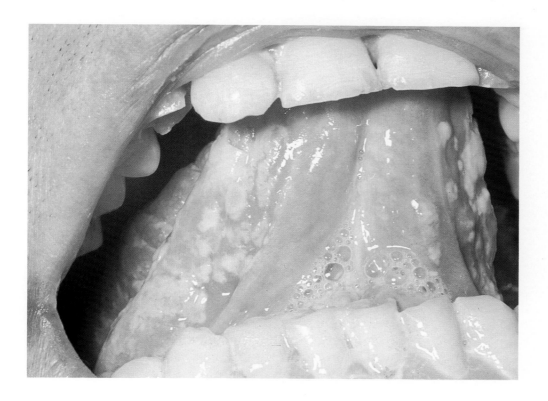

FIGURE 5.24 Oral candidosis. Extensive yellowish-white plaques are visible on both sides of the tongue and on the buccal mucosa.

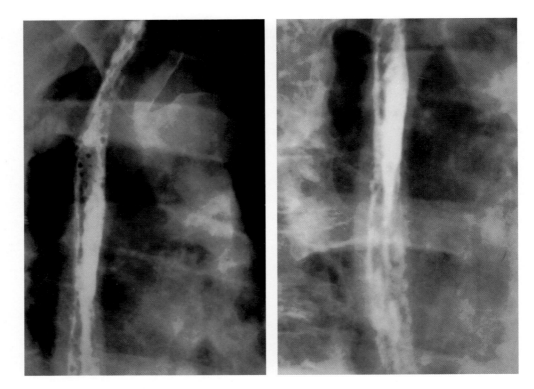

FIGURE 5.25 Oesophageal candidosis: barium swallow. The mucosal outline is irregular and there are many 'filling defects' due to mucosal plaques of candida.

Candida albicans exists in either a yeast phase, when reproduction is by budding, or in a pseudohyphal phase (Fig. 5.26) thought to be associated with pathogenicity.

Candida pneumonia (Fig. 5.27) usually develops late in the course of disseminated (systemic) candidosis (compare aspergillus pneumonia). In these cases the usual portal of entry for *Candida* species is the mouth, oesophagus or lower gastrointestinal tract, or by way of intravenous cannulae used for parenteral nutrition, and spread is by the bloodstream to involve the kidneys, spleen and liver, and later the lungs, pulmonary lesions having the appearance of multiple small abscesses

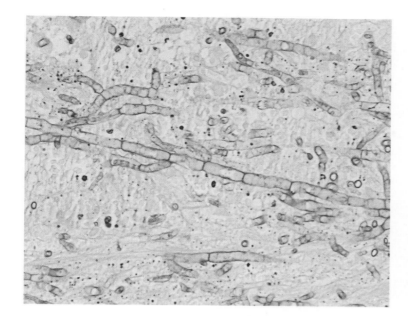

FIGURE 5.26 *Candida albicans* pseudohyphal phase. Long chains of elongated organisms are seen. There is no true branching but budding takes place irregularly at the sides of the chain. Periodic acid–Schiff stain.

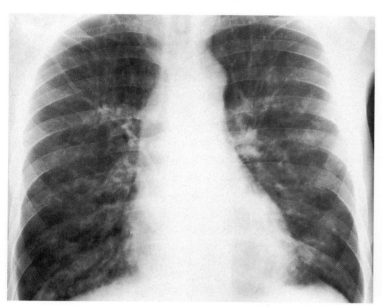

FIGURE 5.27 Candida pneumonia. There is widespread patchy or nodular consolidation, most prominent at the lung bases.

(Fig. 5.28). However, in a proportion of patients with systemic candidosis the lungs or bronchi are the primary portal of entry, usually in those who have a tracheostomy or endotracheal intubation for mechanical ventilation, and who have already received antibacterial agents as well as being immunocompromised.

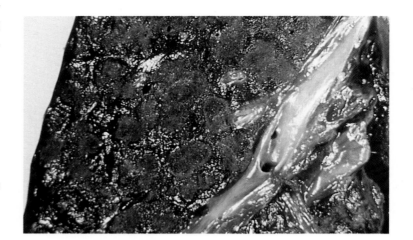

FIGURE 5.28 Candida pneumonia. Numerous nodules are prominent on the cut surface of the right lower lobe of this postmortem specimen from the patient in Fig. 5.27.

CRYPTOCOCCOSIS

Cryptococcus neoformans is a yeast-like fungus that is most easily identified by its thick mucoid capsule (Fig. 5.29).

Pulmonary infection with *C. neoformans* may be clinically silent, particularly when it occurs in an immunologically competent individual. It may then be discovered on a routine chest radiograph as a cryptococcoma (Fig. 5.30). Cryptococcus pneumonia (Fig. 5.31) occurs more frequently in immunocompromised individuals, and there is a particular association with Hodgkin's disease, the precise reason for which is unclear.

Both occult and overt pulmonary infection may be followed by disseminated cryptococcosis, of which meningitis is the most frequently recognized manifestation. Cryptococcal meningitis occurs particularly in chronically immunosuppressed subjects and has an incidence of 2–5% in patients with AIDS. The organism may be identified in the cerebrospinal fluid by negative staining with India ink, the capsule showing up as a clear, unstained area against the dark background of the ink, and also by antigen detection in serum or cerebrospinal fluid. Treatment is with amphotericin B and 5-fluorocytosine, followed by maintenance therapy with fluconazole or itraconazole in AIDS patients with meningitis.

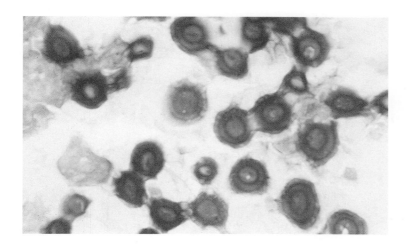

FIGURE 5.29 *Cryptococcus neoformans*. The thick capsule is easily seen in this section from the lung lesions shown in Fig. 5.30. Mucicarmine stain.

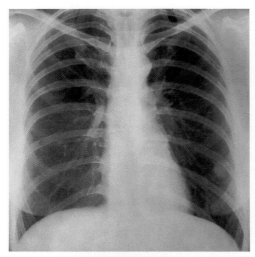

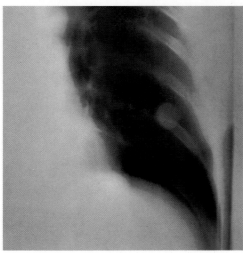

FIGURE 5.30 Cryptococcoma. There is a rounded homogeneous density in the left lower lobe on this routine chest radiograph (upper) in an asymptomatic 37-year-old woman. The tomogram (lower) shows that the opacity lies posteriorly; it does not contain any calcification and has a smooth outline.

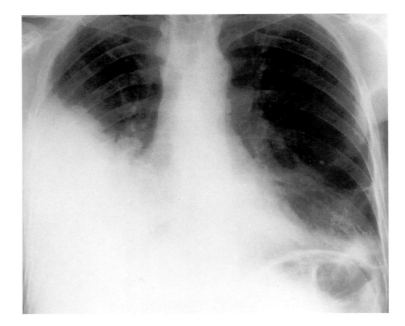

FIGURE 5.31 Cryptococcal pneumonia. There is consolidation of the right middle and lower lobes and at the left lung base. In addition, scattered round densities are present in both lung fields, which may represent old, healed cryptococcosis. The patient had chronic myeloid leukaemia.

HISTOPLASMOSIS

Histoplasma capsulatum is a small yeast that is endemic in eastern central USA; it is found most commonly in soil contaminated by the excreta of birds or bats. The infection may be asymptomatic, leading only to a positive reaction to the histoplasmin intradermal skin test (delayed hypersensitivity, Type IV, reaction). Patients presenting with mild respiratory symptoms may be discovered to have a peripheral infiltrate together with hilar lymphadenopathy (Fig. 5.32), for which treatment is unlikely to be required. Healed lesions may result in a single dense small peripheral shadow on the chest radiograph.

More severe infections may follow heavy exposure to the organism such as may occur during the exploration of caves colonized by bats. An acute bronchopneumonia may then develop (Fig. 5.33); this may heal without treatment but will require intravenous amphotericin B in severe cases. Healing is followed by widespread fibrosis and calcification ('buckshot calcification'), the size and number of the calcified lesions corresponding to the size and number of the original infiltrates (Fig. 5.34). Typical lesions on the chest radiograph are composed of a central calcified core and a surrounding, less dense halo.

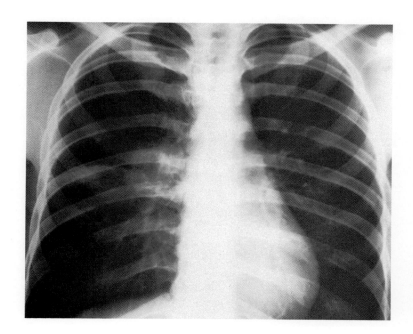

FIGURE 5.32   *Histoplasma capsulatum* primary infection. There is soft shadowing in the right middle lobe and marked right hilar lymphadenopathy.

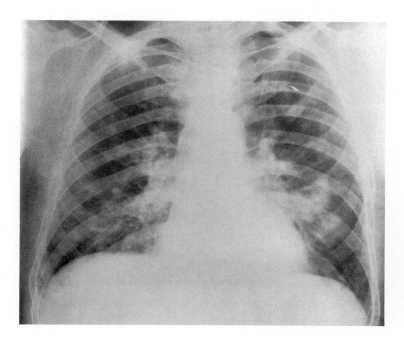

FIGURE 5.33   *Histoplasma capsulatum* bronchopneumonia. Patchy pneumonic lesions are present throughout both lung fields and are most marked in the left lower zone. Healing occurred without antifungal therapy.

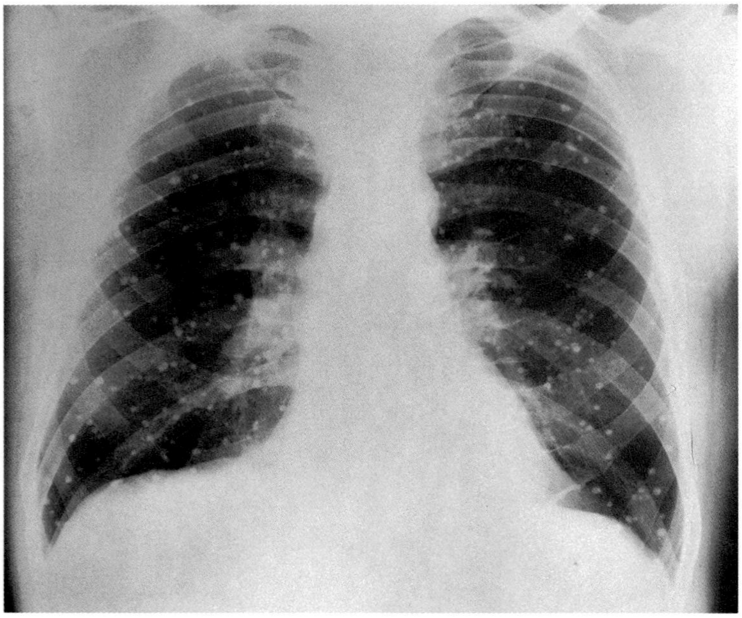

FIGURE 5.34 *Histoplasma capsulatum* 'buckshot calcification'. Chest radiograph of the patient in Fig. 5.33 taken thirteen years later. Widespread nodules are easily seen, many calcified. They are most numerous in the left lower zone where the heaviest shadowing was previously visible.

Inhalation exposure most commonly gives rise to very widespread, medium-sized to small nodular lesions (Fig. 5.35), but may also produce very fine nodular lesions in the granulomatous form of the disease (Fig. 5.36). In most cases of inhalation exposure antifungal therapy is not required.

Acute disseminated histoplasmosis may follow the primary infection and is most frequent in immuno-suppressed patients and in infants. The organism infects the reticuloendothelial system, gastrointestinal tract and lung, in which the appearances may be those of miliary shadowing. Disseminated histoplasmosis is fatal unless treated with amphotericin B.

COCCIDIOIDOMYCOSIS

Coccidioides immitis is a soil-dwelling fungus that is found in the south-western USA and in central parts of South America. The usual route of infection is via the lungs and the diagnosis is made by isolating characteristic spherules, containing endospores, from sputum or biopsy material. Most cases of primary coccidioidomycosis resolve spontaneously and are accompanied by the development of a positive coccidioidin skin test.

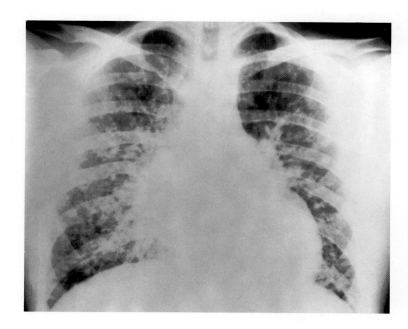

FIGURE 5.35 *Histoplasma capsulatum* bronchopneumonia. These lesions are smaller than those in Fig. 5.33. This is the most common appearance of acute histoplasmosis at presentation.

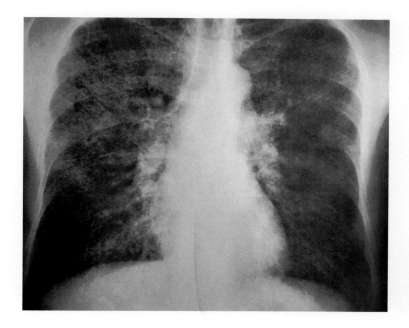

FIGURE 5.36 *Histoplasma capsulatum* granulomatous form. Widespread, very fine nodular shadowing is present throughout both lung fields.

Primary infections may cause hilar lymphadenopathy (Fig. 5.37), patchy opacities in the lung fields or pleural effusions. An inactive lesion may appear as a dense

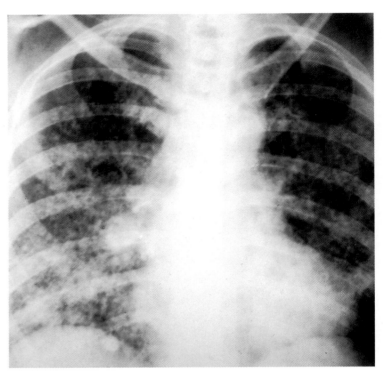

FIGURE 5.37
Coccidioidomycosis. In this primary infection there are small interstitial infiltrates and prominent right hilar and paratracheal lymphadenopathy.

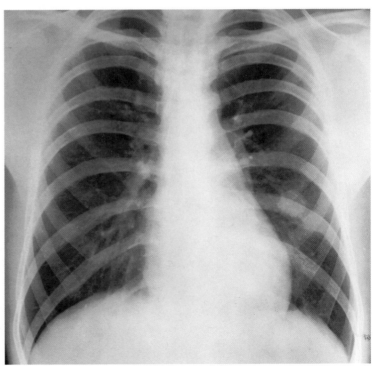

FIGURE 5.38 Coccidioidoma. This routine chest radiograph shows a homogeneous round shadow in the left mid-zone. The coccidioidin skin test was strongly positive.

rounded opacity on the chest radiograph and is termed a coccidioidoma (Fig. 5.38).

Progressive coccidioidomycosis follows the primary infection in about one percent of cases. Progressive disease may take a number of forms, of which the commonest is bronchopneumonia (Fig. 5.39); the healing of such a lesion may result in the formation of a thin-walled or 'eggshell' cavity, which may contain a fluid level (Fig. 5.40). Other forms of progressive coccidioidomycosis include miliary dissemination (Fig. 5.41),

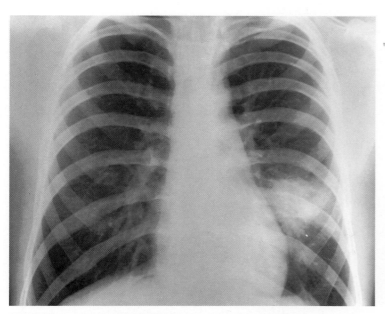

FIGURE 5.39
Coccidioidomycosis. In this chest radiograph of the patient in Fig. 5.38 taken three months later, the shadowing in the left mid-zone has increased in extent and its outline has become poorly defined.

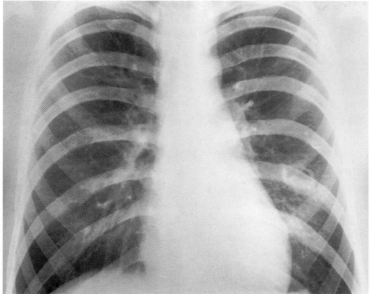

FIGURE 5.40
Coccidioidomycosis. In this chest radiograph of the patient in Fig. 5.39 taken five months later, the area of bronchopneumonia has healed, leaving a typical thin-walled 'eggshell' cavity.

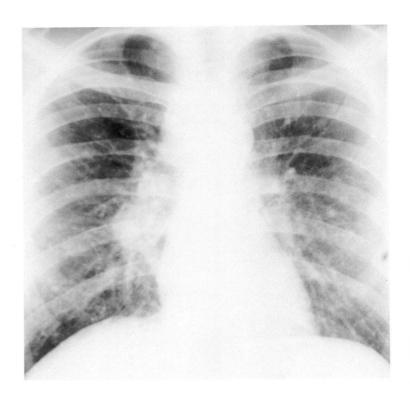

FIGURE 5.41
Coccidioidomycosis. There is
mottling throughout both lung
fields (miliary dissemination),
and right hilar
lymphadenopathy.

which is usually rapidly fatal, and a chronic granulomatous reaction in the lungs (Fig. 5.42), skin, joints,
meninges and brain. Treatment of progressive disease
should be with intravenous amphotericin B.

BLASTOMYCOSIS

Blastomyces dermatitidis is a soil fungus found in the
south-eastern USA. A granulomatous reaction occurs
which most frequently affects the skin and lungs; skin
lesions may be the presenting feature. A mild bronchopneumonia with hilar gland enlargement is frequently
self-limiting (Fig. 5.43), and healing leaves residual
abnormalities on the chest radiograph and a positive
blastomycin skin test.

Pulmonary involvement is usually part of a systemic
disease, which may involve the genitourinary and central
nervous systems, and there may be miliary shadowing
on the chest radiograph. Massive opacities in the lungs

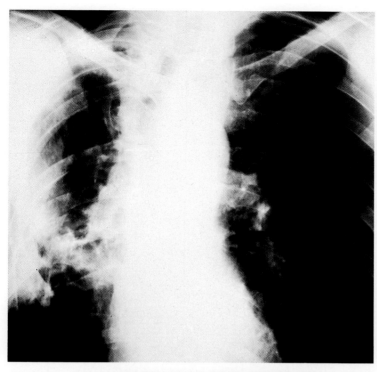

FIGURE 5.42
Coccidioidomycosis: granulomatous form. There is extensive fibrous scarring with loss of volume and multiple thin-walled cavities in the right upper and middle lobes.

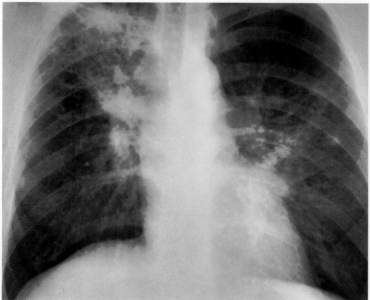

FIGURE 5.43 Blastomycosis. Bronchopneumonia affects the right upper lobe and apical left lower lobe. On the right there has been loss of volume with cavitation.

may cavitate, the cavities frequently persisting after treatment (Fig. 5.44).

The diagnosis is made by finding the fungus in biopsy material, and treatment is with systemic amphotericin B, or ketoconazole in milder cases without CNS involvement.

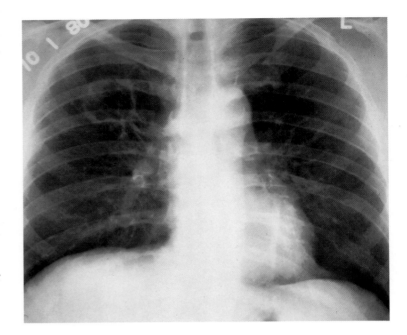

FIGURE 5.44 Blastomycosis. A cavity persists in the right upper lobe after successful treatment with amphotericin B for subacute pneumonia.

PNEUMOCYSTIS CARINII PNEUMONIA

Pneumocystis carinii is a protozoon that may be found as a commensal in the upper respiratory tract. In immuno-compromised patients the organism may become invasive and cause a widespread interstitial pneumonia. In the past, this occurred most frequently in patients with acute lymphoblastic leukaemia or lymphoma who had received prolonged cytotoxic chemotherapy and corticosteroids (Fig. 5.45). Oral co-trimoxazole, given to these patients during remission induction, has proved to be highly effective prophylaxis. The organism has assumed greater importance again with the increasing incidence of the acquired immune deficiency syndrome (AIDS).

There is frequently a history of coryza or a sore throat for a few days before the onset of marked tachypnoea and cyanosis. There is usually a fever of up to 40°C, but comparatively little systemic toxicity or distress in relation to the severity of the hypoxia and tachypnoea. In individuals without AIDS but who have received high doses of corticosteroids, the time of the initial manifestation of the illness is most often during the reduction of corticosteroid dosage. In individuals with AIDS pneumocystis pneumonia (PCP) has become one of the classical presenting and diagnostic features.

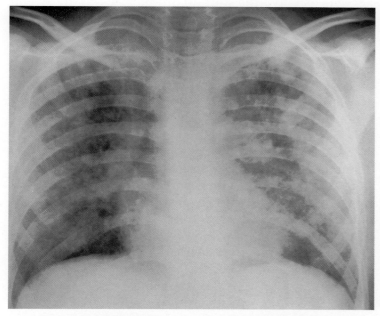

FIGURE 5.45 *Pneumocystis carinii* pneumonia. There is bilateral dense interstitial shadowing. This 8-year-old boy had received two years of maintenance chemotherapy for acute lymphoblastic leukaemia.

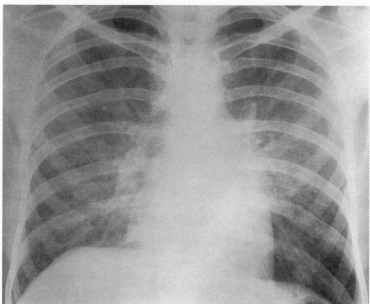

FIGURE 5.46 *Pneumocystis carinii* pneumonia. Interstitial shadowing is much finer in texture than in Fig. 5.45, and there is relative sparing of the lung apices and of the left lower lobe.

Pneumocystis carinii gives rise to an interstitial pneumonia with a copious alveolar exudate, and the chest radiograph shows widespread interstitial shadowing, frequently with an air bronchogram. Sometimes there is sparing of one or more lobes of the lung (Fig. 5.46). *Pneumocystis carinii* pneumonia has to be distinguished from viral infections which also produce an interstitial pneumonia, and from adult respiratory distress syndrome ('shock lung').

There is usually little sputum production but the alveoli are filled with a proteinaceous exudate which has a foamy appearance in histological sections (Fig. 5.47) and contains the cysts from which the organism derives its name (Fig. 5.48). The diagnosis is made most reliably by biopsy, which is most convenient using the trans-bronchial method through a fibreoptic bronchoscope. When this is combined with broncho-alveolar lavage, the diagnosis can be made in 100% of patients.

Treatment should be with high-dosage co-trimoxazole (trimethoprim 16mg plus sulphamethoxazole 80mg per kilogram of body weight per day) which should be given intravenously since gastrointestinal absorption may be poor in these ill patients. Symptomatic improvement is usually rapid in non-AIDS patients but may take longer in those with AIDS. In all cases several days may elapse before clearing of the exudate and of the chest radiograph. If co-trimoxazole fails, then penta-midine 4mg/kg/day is used, or, if not tolerated, dapsone plus trimethoprim, clindamycin plus primaquine, or trimetrexate may be tried. Secondary prophylaxis with monthly nebulized pentamidine or with co-trimoxazole is given to AIDS patients.

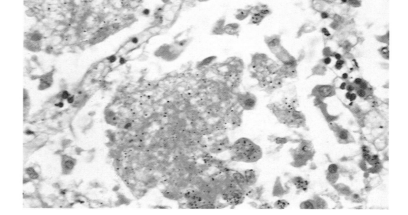

FIGURE 5.47 *Pneumocystis carinii* pneumonia. This open lung biopsy specimen shows a typical foamy proteinaceous exudate in the alveoli. Haematoxylin and eosin stain.

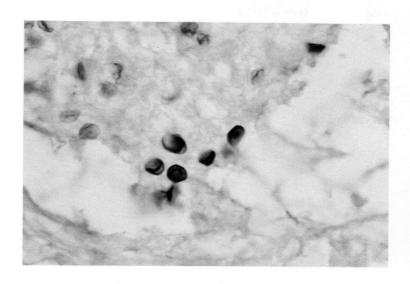

FIGURE 5.48 *Pneumocystis carinii* pneumonia. In the same open lung biopsy from the patient in Fig. 5.47, the cysts have stained darkly; they are seen intact at the periphery of the exudate, and rather fragmented at its centre. Grocott stain.

Chapter 6

Differential Diagnosis Treatment and Complications

DIFFERENTIAL DIAGNOSIS

The history is important, as bacterial pneumonias are usually of more sudden onset than those of non-bacterial origin. The patient may give a history of travelling in an area endemic for histoplasma or coccidioides, and details of other diseases and immunosuppressive drugs are important.

In all cases where sputum is available it should be examined for aerobic and anaerobic bacteria, acid-fast bacilli and fungi. In recent years the use of gas–liquid chromatography (Fig. 6.1), which shows a profile of fatty acids produced by anaerobic metabolism, has aided the diagnosis of anaerobic infections. Routine cultures for viruses, mycoplasma and rickettsias are not yet available. The white blood count is high in bacterial pneumonias, but may be normal in pneumonia due to viruses or mycoplasma. Blood cultures may be positive early in the illness, particularly in cases of pneumonia due

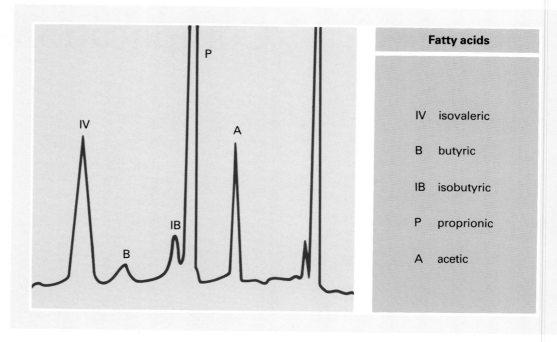

Fatty acids
IV   isovaleric
B   butyric
IB   isobutyric
P   proprionic
A   acetic

FIGURE 6.1   Gas–liquid chromatograph of the sputum of a patient with a lung abscess due to *Bacteroides fragilis*. The peaks indicate fatty acids. The profile of fatty acids produced by anaerobic metabolism is characteristic for a given anaerobe.

to *Streptococcus pneumoniae*. A four-fold rising titre of antibodies in the serum confirms the diagnosis of viral, rickettsial or mycoplasmal pneumonia. Cold agglutinins are frequently found in the sera in cases of mycoplasma pneumonia. Autoantibodies which agglutinate human red blood cells at 4°C develop in the sera of over half the patients with *Mycoplasma pneumoniae* during the second week of illness. Toxoplasmosis may be diagnosed using the Sabin–Feldmann dye test. If the patient has a pleural effusion this should be aspirated and a pleural biopsy performed using Abram's needle. In infections due to *Aspergillus fumigatus*, *Histoplasma capsulatum* or *Coccidioides immitis*, skin tests can be helpful.

In some cases of severe pneumonia, particularly in immunosuppressed hosts, it may be necessary to perform a lung biopsy using a drill or open procedure to obtain a sample of lung tissue. This will enable the correct diagnosis to be made and the correct treatment to be instigated.

Radiological Appearance

Radiological appearances in patients with pneumonia are very varied. Lobar consolidation without shrinkage may be seen, as may widespread bilateral foci of consolidation. Local areas of consolidation are more common in bacterial pneumonia than in those of other aetiology. Abscesses are more commonly seen in pneumonia due to *Staphylococcus pyogenes*, *Klebsiella pneumoniae* and anaerobes, whilst *Mycobacterium tuberculosis* pneumonia typically cavitates. In some cases, miliary shadows, atelectasis and pleural effusion will be found. In all cases of pneumonia, a chest radiograph should be taken when the patient has recovered clinically to make sure that there is no residual pathology.

Physiology

In the early stages of pneumonia, the affected part of the lung is perfused with blood but is not ventilated with air as the alveoli are full of fluid. There is therefore a right-to-left shunt and, in consequence, a fall in the arterial oxygen level. If this is severe, the patient becomes cyanosed and delirious. Unless the patient has pre-existing lung disease, hyperventilation will prevent carbon dioxide retention. If the extent of the pneumonia is extensive, the patient will go into hypoxic type 1 respiratory failure. In chronic bronchitics, however, the arterial carbon dioxide level may rise and extensive pneumonia may cause type 2 respiratory failure, that is, hypoxia with carbon dioxide retention.

Carcinoma Presenting as Pneumonia

In patients who have been smokers it must always be remembered that pneumonia may be distal to a carcinoma causing obstruction in the bronchial tree (Fig. 6.2). All patients recovering from pneumonia should have a chest radiograph six weeks after all symptoms have disappeared to make sure that there is no underlying pathology, such as carcinoma.

Allergic, Chemical and Physical Causes of Pneumonitis

An allergic reaction to *A. fumigatus* can cause 'flitting' pulmonary shadows (Fig. 6.3). This is accompanied by

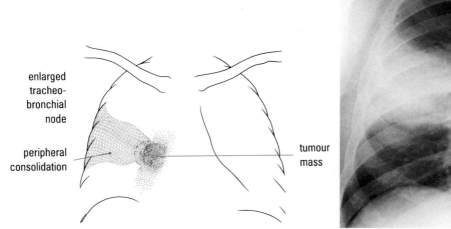

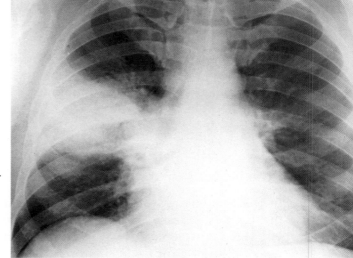

FIGURE 6.2 Pneumonia distal to carcinoma. There is a segmental area of opacification in the right middle zone with a density at the right hilum. No air bronchogram is present.

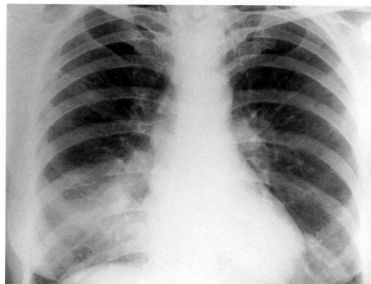

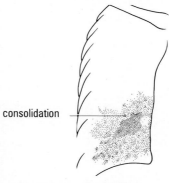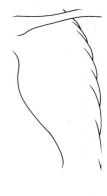

consolidation

FIGURE 6.3a *Aspergillus fumigatus* pneumonia. A triangular opacity adjacent to the right hilum represents an area of consolidation. The patient had ABPA with blood eosinophilia, a positive skin-prick test and serum precipitins to *A. fumigatus*.

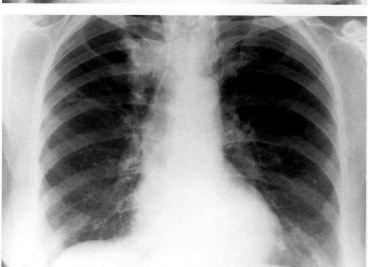

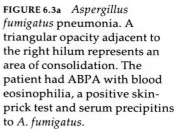

fresh opacity

FIGURE 6.3b The opacity cleared, but a fresh ill-defined opacity occurred in the upper right zone.

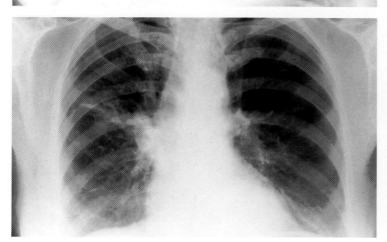

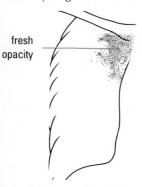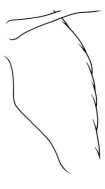

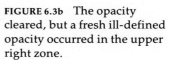

cone-shaped opacity

FIGURE 6.3c The opacity in **b** cleared, but a cone-shaped density developed in the right middle zone.

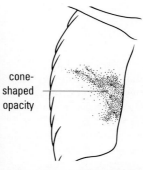

blood eosinophilia (Fig. 6.4) and a positive immediate skin test to *A. fumigatus*. The pulmonary lesions respond to corticosteroids.

Lipoid pneumonia may result from the aspiration of

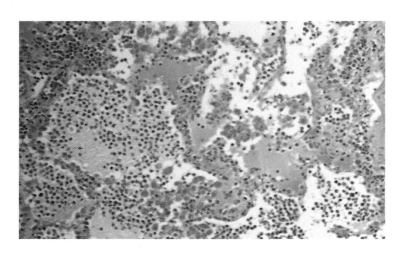

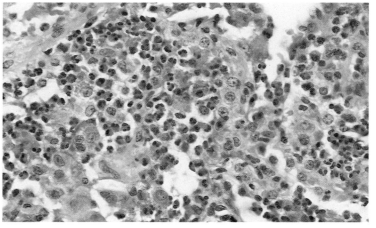

FIGURE 6.4 Eosinophilic pneumonia. The low-power view shows cellular filling of the alveoli; higher magnification shows that virtually all the free cells are eosinophils. Such an allergic pneumonia may be due to fungi, drugs or metazoan parasites passing through the lungs, or may be cryptogenic. Haematoxylin and eosin stain.

oils, taken in nasal drops or as an aperient (Figs 6.5 and 6.6). Aspiration pneumonia may also be due to oesophageal disease (Fig. 6.7). Inhalation of vomit (Figs 6.8 and 6.9), which usually occurs when consciousness

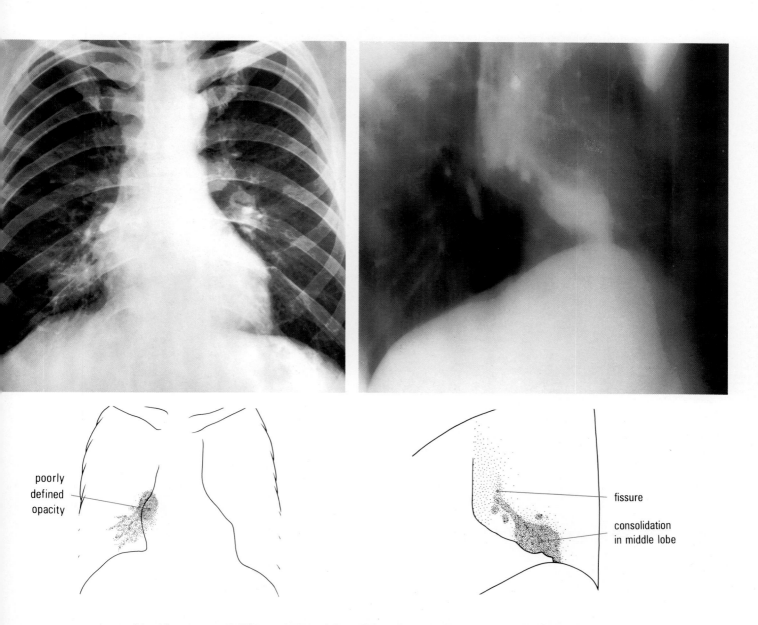

FIGURE 6.5 Lipoid pneumonia. This patient took liquid paraffin regularly last thing at night. A 4cm poorly defined opacity is present in the right middle lobe, where it might easily be mistaken for a carcinoma.

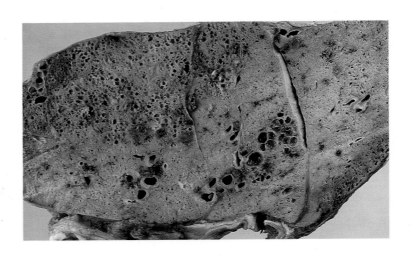

FIGURE 6.6 Exogenous lipoid pneumonia. There is diffuse yellow consolidation. Unknown to medical attendants, the patient had been ingesting, and inadvertently aspirating, massive amounts of liquid paraffin because of constipation. Courtesy of Dr R. Salm.

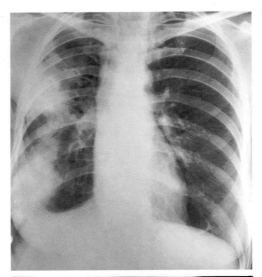

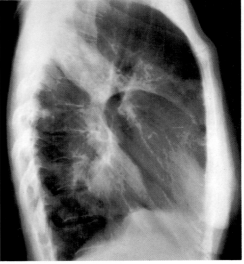

FIGURE 6.7 Aspiration pneumonia due to achalasia. Ill-defined areas of opacification are present in the anterior and posterior segments of the right upper lobe and right lower lobe. The gastric air bubble is absent and the mediastinum has a straight right border due to a dilated oesophagus.

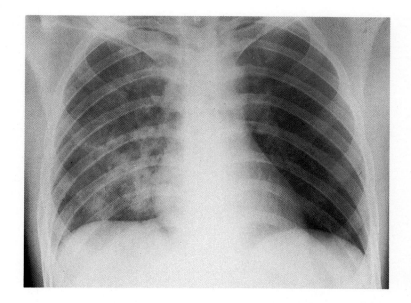

FIGURE 6.8 Right-sided inhalation pneumonia.

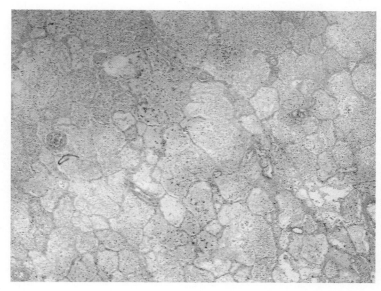

FIGURE 6.9 Inhalation of gastric contents. The alveoli are flooded by a haemorrhagic oedema. The brownish discoloration is due to the action of hydrochloric acid on haemoglobin. Haematoxylin and eosin stain. Courtesy of Dr W.R. Geddie.

is impaired, may cause widespread pneumonia. This is due to gastric acid being inhaled into the lungs, and may be associated with infection by a mixed population of bacteria including anaerobes. Treatment is with antibiotics and corticosteroids. Irradiation (Fig. 6.10) and inhalation of a variety of irritant gases (Fig. 6.11) may also cause pneumonitis.

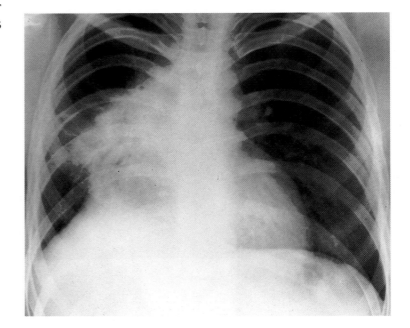

FIGURE 6.10 Radiation pneumonitis. There is a poorly defined extensive area of opacification blending with the right side of the mediastinum. Note the air bronchogram; the patient had been treated by radiotherapy for pulmonary metastases from a teratoma of the testis.

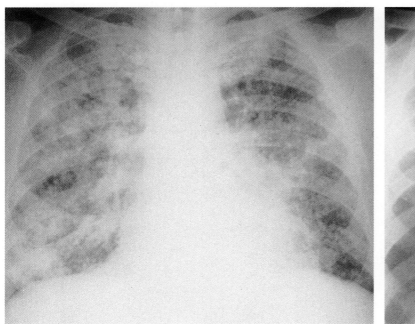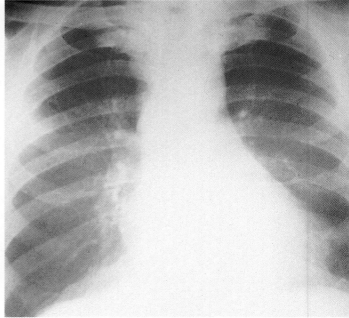

FIGURE 6.11 Pneumonitis following inhalation of nitric acid fumes. Widespread shadowing indicates patchy consolidation in both lungs (left), with the right side affected more severely than the left. After two months (right) the lungs are virtually clear but are overinflated and there is some reduction in vascularity on both sides, suggesting some residual obstruction of the airways.

It is important to make an accurate diagnosis so that the correct antibiotic treatment may be instigated. In severely ill patients, however, it may be necessary to start treatment while waiting for results of bacteriological investigations. In life-threatening infections it is often important to commence treatment with antibiotics active against Gram-positive, Gram-negative, aerobic and anaerobic organisms until bacterial confirmation of the diagnosis is obtained. A suitable combination of antibiotics to cover the most likely pathogens might be benzylpenicillin, flucloxacillin, gentamicin and metronidazole. Another possibility would be one of the cephalosporins, such as cefotaxime or cefuroxime, with flucloxacillin and an aminoglycoside. If the patient is allergic to penicillin, erythromycin can be used instead. When a specific pathogen has been isolated, the appropriate antibiotic is given and the others stopped.

Attention to general measures such as rehydration and analgesia are important. If the patient is hypoxic, humidified oxygen should be given. If there are significant secretions then physiotherapy is indicated. In some patients with severe life-threatening pneumonia, artificial ventilation will be required. Complications should be treated as appropriate.

Failure to Respond to Treatment

If a patient with pneumonia fails to respond to treatment one must ask, 'Is the diagnosis correct?' The physical signs of pulmonary embolus or pleural effusion may sometimes mimic those of pneumonia. If the diagnosis of pneumonia is correct, has one identified the causative agent? Sputum must be examined for acid-fast bacilli, fungi and anaerobes. It may be necessary to proceed to fibreoptic bronchoscopy with aspiration of secretions to obtain better samples of bronchial secretions for bacteriological analysis. If there is any suspicion that the patient may have local bronchial obstruction due to stricture, carcinoma or foreign body, a bronchoscopy must be performed. In patients who are immunosuppressed, as a result of disease or therapy, unusual pathogens such as *Pneumocystis carinii* should be suspected.

COMPLICATIONS

Most cases of pneumonia, diagnosed accurately and treated properly, will resolve without complications. However, the following complications may occur in certain cases: pleural effusions, lung abscesses (Fig. 6.12), empyema (Figs 6.13 and 6.14), atelectasis, gangrene (Fig. 6.15) and postpneumonic fibrosis (Fig. 6.16). In severe pneumonia, respiratory failure or cor pulmonale may occur, particularly if the patient has pre-existing respiratory disease. Other important, but fortunately

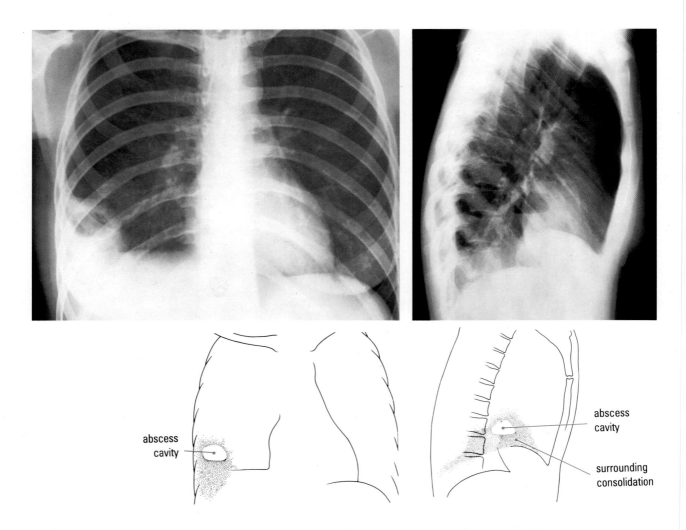

FIGURE 6.12 Lung abscess complicating pneumonia. Thin-walled ring shadows with air fluid levels are present in the right lower lobe.

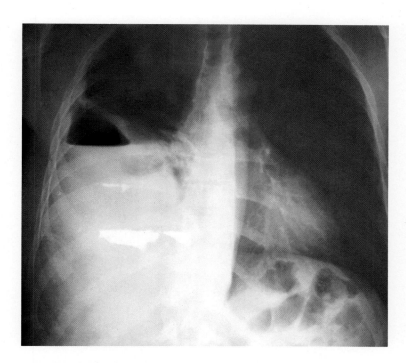

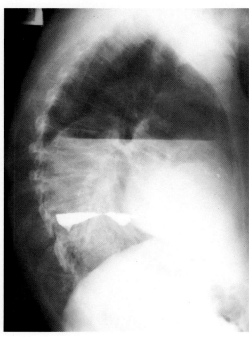

FIGURE 6.13 Empyema and pyopneumothorax. Lipiodol has been injected into the cavity to show its lower limit. The underlying lung is partly collapsed.

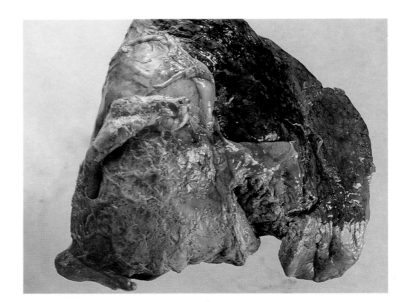

FIGURE 6.14 Empyema. The posterior surface of the lung is covered by a shaggy, fibrinopurulent exudate.

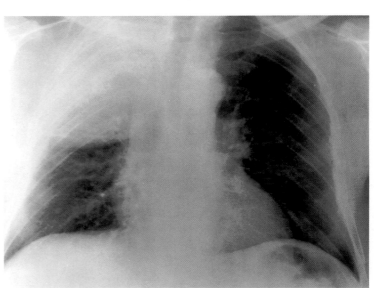

FIGURE 6.15 Gangrene in the right upper lobe following pneumonia.

rare, complications are septicaemia, meningitis, jaundice, myocarditis, pericarditis, thromboembolic phenomena, pneumothorax, haemolytic anaemia and glomerulonephritis. A common, but not serious, association of infections with *Streptococcus pneumoniae* is herpes labialis.

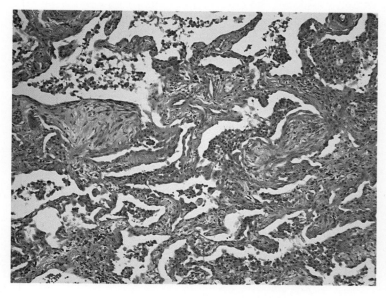

FIGURE 6.16 Postpneumonic fibrosis. Micropolypoid knots of granulation tissue, rich in ground substance (Masson bodies), protrude into the alveoli. Haematoxylin and eosin stain.

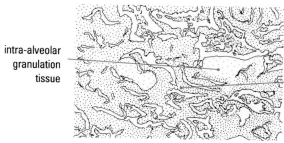

intra-alveolar granulation tissue

alveolar wall

Lung Abscesses

A lung abscess is most frequently produced by bacterial infection but there may be other causes, such as pulmonary infarction and carcinoma of the bronchus. Lung abscesses may follow bacterial pneumonia, particularly pneumonia due to *Staphylococcus pyogenes* (see Fig. 2.4), *Klebsiella pneumoniae*, *Mycobacterium tuberculosis* or anaerobes (see Figs 2.8 and 2.9). They may also be associated with aspiration of vomit, infected teeth and sinuses, chronic bronchitis or bronchiectasia and post-operative states. Very ill or debilitated patients and those with neuromuscular disease are particularly at risk. A lung abscess may follow aspiration of a foreign body. The patient will present with copious purulent sputum and chest radiography will show a cavity, often with a fluid level. A further complication is pyopneumothorax. If there is any suggestion of bronchial obstruction in a patient with lung abscess, a bronchoscopy must be performed. Treatment is by physiotherapy with postural drainage and a prolonged course of antibiotics. Surgery is occasionally required.

Index